PROSTATE CANCER
SHEEP OR WOLF?

MURRAY KEITH WADSWORTH

NAVIGATING SYSTEMIC MISINFORMATION

FOREWORD BY DR. CAROLE WYATT

PROSTATE CANCER: SHEEP OR WOLF?

To contact the author, submit your request at **http://sheeporwolfcancer.com**

Every effort has been made to trace and contact all applicable copyright holders prior to publication. If there are any inadvertent omissions or errors, the author will be pleased to correct these at the earliest opportunity.

Print edition ISBN: 978-1-7329381-0-6
E-book edition ISBN: 978-1-7329381-1-3

The stories of the men named in the prologue are real, each known to the author. To protect their privacy certain details have been excluded and their real names have been replaced with pseudonyms.

This book is about the author's medical journey with prostate cancer. The reader is advised that the author is not a medical doctor nor medically trained. The book does not provide medical, psychological, financial, or other professional advice or services, and it is not intended nor should be considered a substitute for professional medical advice, diagnosis, or treatment. If you are in need of expert medical advice or assistance, you should seek it from a source or physician of your choice. Never disregard professional medical advice or delay seeking professional medical advice because of something you have read in this book. The entire contents of this book, including text, graphics, images, and information obtained from other sources reflect the author's experiences and opinions, and are for informational purposes only. Although the author shares his experiences and opinions regarding specific tests, physicians, institutions, products, and procedures, no recommendations of any kind are suggested or offered. The author has not received any remuneration for mentioning any tests, physicians, institutions, products, or procedures. The author's references are provided for informational purposes only and do not constitute endorsement of any website or other sources. Readers are further advised that the website URLs listed in this book may change, as they did while the manuscript was being written. Reliance on any information provided by the author in this book is solely at your own risk.

Edited by Stacey Donovan
Cover artwork and other illustrations by Helen Lucy Studio
Author photograph by Maggie Messer Photography
Publishing services by AuthorImprints

In fond memory of Joerg Groessler, 1952–2007.
Our friendship and mutual business respect took me to England.

And gratefulness beyond words for
my daughter, Shannon, my son, Matthew,
and my closest friends.
Their support is shared within.

2016 RV JOURNEY

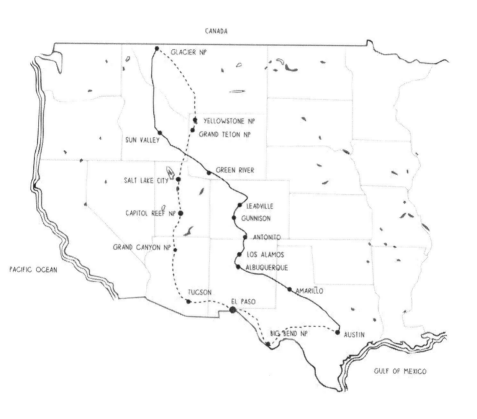

CANADA

GLACIER NP

YELLOWSTONE NP
GRAND TETON NP

SUN VALLEY

GREEN RIVER

SALT LAKE CITY

LEADVILLE
GUNNISON

CAPITOL REEF NP

ANTONITO

LOS ALAMOS
ALBUQUERQUE

GRAND CANYON NP

PACIFIC OCEAN

TUCSON

AMARILLO

EL PASO

BIG BEND NP

AUSTIN

GULF OF MEXICO

——————— OUTBOUND PATH
------------- RETURN PATH

NP - NATIONAL PARK
FOR REFERENCE, NOT DRAWN TO EXACT SCALE

CONTENTS

List of Graphs

FOREWORD

Is Prostate Cancer the New Breast Cancer?

Anyone who loves to ski will know how interesting chairlift conversations can be. Even with a total stranger you are already bonded by your passion for the mountains, and something about the experience can bring a depth of disclosure you would not normally begin to contemplate in any other setting. Perhaps it is something to do with sitting side by side, with no awkward eye contact. If the lift is a long one, you quickly get beyond "Where are you from?" and "What do you do?" Keith and I met on a ski trip, in the beautiful Swiss resort of Flims, organized by the Ski Club of Great Britain—part of their "Peak Experience" program (in other words, for over-fifties!). I learned that he was from Austin, Texas, and had been running a "very small" IT business in Surrey after its previous owner died tragically young. Keith was divorced and had brought up two children alone, the younger with profound disabilities. In return I told him I was a doctor, also divorced and effectively a single parent, with twenty years of experience as a general physician, then ten years as a breast cancer specialist working largely in breast cancer diagnostics and genetics. A few days into the trip, Keith shared with me that he had recently been diagnosed with prostate cancer.

I dealt with this kind of thing every day, so I wasn't taken aback or lost for words. At the end of the trip we exchanged contact details, and over the next few weeks and months I researched everything I could about prostate cancer. There were many similarities between breast cancer and prostate cancer in the United Kingdom, but also fundamental differences. Citing Cancer Research UK:[1]

Some Similarities

- Breast cancer is the most common cancer in the United Kingdom (55,122 new cases in 2015 and affecting one in eight women) while prostate cancer is a close second (47,151 new cases in 2015 and affecting one in eight men).
- Almost half (46 percent) of female breast cancer cases each year are diagnosed in females aged sixty-five and over; more than half (54 percent) of prostate cancer cases each year are diagnosed in males aged seventy and over.
- Surgery for both breast and prostate cancer has far-reaching effects on well-being, lifestyle, and sexuality.

But, as Keith will point out in this book, statistics are of little use to an individual patient; a common example of this is BMI—body mass index—commonly used both in the United Kingdom and the United States to assess weight-related health risks. But BMI was never intended to be used for *individuals*—it was developed by Adolphe Quetelet in the early nineteenth century to study what he called "social physics" and the health of populations. And similarly, looking at another statement from Cancer Research UK, *"More than eight in ten (84 percent) men diagnosed with prostate cancer in England and Wales survive their disease for ten years or more"* is meaningless on an individual scale unless we have some way of knowing who will comprise the two in ten who *don't* survive for ten years or more.

Some cases of breast cancer (especially the variety known as *in situ breast carcinoma*, where the cancer cells are completely contained and have not grown into surrounding breast tissue) would likewise sometimes not result in significant disease. Similarly, many cases of prostate cancer never progress to a degree that would have an impact on quality of life or life expectancy. In both cases however, our current knowledge does not allow us to clearly distinguish the cases that will. Here in the United Kingdom, for the past couple of years, use of the genetic profiling test Oncotype DX has become more widespread—not to decide if a woman needs treatment or not, but whether she will benefit from harsh and costly chemotherapy treatment following surgery. More developments are sure to follow which will allow us to stratify risks even further.

But the Differences

- There is intense public awareness of breast cancer, with constant media attention. In the United Kingdom, the press contains articles daily about new research, treatment innovations, celebrities diagnosed with breast cancer, and so on. Massive charity funding is raised every year; with everything "pink" drawing huge public support. Prostate cancer barely features, and most people could not think of a single male celebrity known to have suffered from the disease, whereas they could easily name at least a dozen well-known women with breast cancer. And it is not that fewer high-profile men suffer; men affected include Robert De Niro, Ryan O'Neal, Harry Belafonte, Governor Jerry Brown, former secretary of state Colin Powell, and the British actors Roger Moore and Ian McKellen.

- Prostate cancer treatment seems to be in the place where breast cancer treatment was an entire generation ago— radical surgery "to be on the safe side," and few options for more conservative approaches.

- The youngest-onset cases of breast cancer are significantly earlier than those of prostate cancer—deaths from breast cancer can and do occur in the twenties and early thirties, meaning that these women die leaving young children and with largely unlived lives. The latest breast cancer mortality data available for the United Kingdom shows an average of 234 deaths per year in women under forty, and 1,152 deaths in women under fifty, compared with one death in men under forty from prostate cancer, and just twenty-two in men under fifty.

Furthermore, there are major differences between the UK and the US approach to treatment. The vast majority of British people are treated for both breast and prostate cancer under the National Health Service (NHS)—which is free at the point of delivery, though overall funding from central government is limited. This means that, because of the economics involved, UK doctors are keen to avoid unnecessary tests or treatment, but nonetheless achieve outcomes as good as anywhere in the world, as published research testifies. Furthermore, UK doctors are generally salaried, and are paid the same regardless of how many surgeries or treatments they provide. When I visited Keith in Austin in October 2015, I was taken aback by the advertising of medical services on radio, on billboards on the highway, in glossy brochures depicting caring happy couples sharing their journey together. My impression is that choosing a treatment path in the United States is actually a lonely and largely unguided journey. In the United Kingdom, all NHS-diagnosed cancer cases have a multidisciplinary evaluation—for breast patients this will involve surgeons, radiologists, pathologists, and oncologists all discussing each case together—at least once, sometimes several times. This ensures that all reasonable options are considered, and provides a high degree of consistency and adherence to best-practice guidance.

Aspects of the Management of Breast Cancer that Would Improve that of Prostate Cancer

I believe that more needs to be done to differentiate between indolent, slow-growing cases of prostate cancer, and aggressive, no-symptoms-until-it's-too-late tumors. This will mean that US health agencies must readily accept novel biological tests such as Oncotype DX. Breast cancer treatment is currently personalized according to a growing list of these biological indicators, with more to come, and prostate cancer treatment must surely follow suit.

Radiological imaging with mammography, ultrasound, and sometimes magnetic resonance imaging (MRI), is a fundamental step in the diagnostic pathway for breast cancer, and is used to guide the biopsy tissue sample to the site of clinical concern. This is rarely the case in prostate cancer, where blood screening concerns are generally followed by random biopsies. Side effects of a biopsy can include bleeding and infection. However, a recent UK study led by Professor Mark Emberton and Dr. Hashim Ahmed from University College London,[2] found that MRI before a first biopsy would allow a large group of the men who are currently referred for biopsy to avoid it. In the study,

MRI alone, without the invasive procedure of taking a tissue sample, was sufficient to rule out safely the possibility of significant prostate cancer. "Taking a random biopsy from the breast would not be accepted, but we accept that in prostate," Dr. Ahmed told the British Broadcasting Corporation.[3]

When I was a junior doctor on a surgical team in 1986, radical mastectomy less than a week from diagnosis was not uncommon. This procedure entailed having everything removed: the breast, the underlying muscle, all accessible lymph nodes—it was always disfiguring, often with horrific side effects. Brave surgeons and even braver patients gradually started removing less and less tissue—the whole breast, maybe, but not the muscle. Subsequently, lumpectomy became widespread practice for smaller tumors, backed up with increasingly precise radiotherapy as a precaution against residual diseased cells. Around ten years ago, techniques were developed to identify the first few lymph nodes in the chain responsible for the cancerous cells, and to remove those but leave the others.

We need much clearer information about treatment options; not scare-mongering tactics, not pushy marketing, but a clear understanding of the facts, the symptoms (or lack of them), and the optimum testing modalities. We need open, honest discussion. My hope is that, driven by men like Keith who are demanding better access to a full range of information about diagnostic and treatment options, the treatment of prostate cancer will soon be managed with the same precision and sensitivity as breast cancer.

Dr. Carole Wyatt

Breast cancer physician, retired, Norfolk, UK

FIVE GUYS

A ndrew was a fit guy in his late fifties when his prostate biopsy was reported to show cancer, a few months ahead of my own diagnosis. He elected surgery for treatment. His prostate, sexual nerves, and multiple lymph nodes were removed. The final diagnosis was downgraded—Andrew did not have prostate cancer.

George travels internationally for his work, well into his seventies. These days he packs a suitcase full of men's diapers for urinary incontinence. Prior to his surgery he understood few details of his diagnosis.

Joe proudly wore his veteran's hat to radiotherapy. My session followed his. Each morning we acknowledged our circumstances with at least a friendly greeting. His diagnosis came to light during an extensive physical checkup following a heart attack. Surgery was scheduled, with seemingly little evaluation of relative risks. The operating urologist found that the lymph nodes contained metastasized cancer, so the prostatectomy was abandoned. Joe was offered radiotherapy to slow the cancer and the onset of symptoms. His disease was deemed incurable.

Peter is a businessman in England. I recognized the Prostate Cancer UK charity awareness pin, a black-and-white enamel male figure, on his lapel. Rather than treating his prostate cancer straightaway, Peter is in a medically supervised monitoring program (aka active surveillance). He was not aware of the risk profile of his tumor cells.

I, Keith, a fit weekend triathlete from Austin, Texas, included healthy checkups as part of my wellness plan. At age forty-seven, a seemingly routine screening for prostate health presented a frightening cancer scare. A biopsy was done. Thankfully it was benign, no cancer, no concerns. At fifty-seven, while living in England, screening raised a second scare, albeit less frightening than the first. But that had a different outcome. Back home in Austin, the biopsy tested positive for prostate cancer. My long-established urologist opened his diary and offered me an appointment for surgery, a radical prostatectomy the following week. Confused, uncertain, and afraid, I felt my life and lifestyle were on the line. Despite the cancer, I followed my instinct to say no. I returned to England in search of answers to my many questions.

INTRODUCTION

As I strive to survive this disease, or at least delay my death from it, I ponder how other men navigate all the confusing information about what is best to do and when to do it. Despite having considerable clinical evidence on this disease, we lack far more. And it seems competing and vested commercial interests contribute to the confusion.

At my young age I resent the perspective, intended it seems as a consolation, a very poor one, that we should accept living with this disease because something else might come along and kill us anyway; say texting while driving or another illness. And I cannot find solace in the common proclamation that if a man lives long enough he will develop prostate cancer, but not die from it.

My story shares my medical experiences and my research efforts in America and Europe before I made my multiple treatment decisions. In my research I found a seemingly infinite number of resources. One that I relied heavily upon was *Prostate Disorders: Your Annual Guide to Prevention, Diagnosis, and Treatment, a US publication.*[4]

The reality of navigating my way through prostate cancer was, and remains, a harsh and challenging journey between hope and fear. Decisions hinge as much, and possibly more, upon the fears of overtreatment and side effects than on the risks of the cancer itself. Much is written about these fears. One provocative source I found in my early efforts of web surfing was the article "Epidemic of Overtreatment of Prostate Cancer Must Stop," published in 2014 by CNN Health, written by Dr. Otis Brawley.[5] I now view such perspectives as contributing to the confusing misinformation. Shouldn't the emphasis be on finding and treating the cancers that kill men?

Throughout my multiple treatment decisions my awareness and efforts focused on key questions. How aggressive is the cancer? Where is all of it? Can it all be removed or killed? If not, can its spread be slowed?

Getting answers to those questions was challenging and confusing. I was surprised by the varying diagnostic methods, medical opinions, and treatment options. Then what does one do with all the messaging that emphasizes finding the best care, and that one's survival outcome is dependent on the skill of the treatment provider and the treatment facility itself? Who would want anything less than the best? And what of the patients who receive far less?

Add to these challenges the cancer-centric marketing messages that bombard us in America. One radio commercial I heard all too often used the tagline—"*Then you learn your cancer is back.*" I came to see this as misinformation, a marketing ploy, or perhaps an exploitation of the challenges with achieving treatment success.

Although the intent of curative treatment is to remove or kill every cancer cell, it is not scientifically possible to prove that all the cancer is gone. The best we can hope for is that the cancer can no longer be detected. When cancer is detected after a perceived curative treatment, the common medical term is *biochemical recurrence*. This outcome is often characterized as the cancer coming back. From my perspective as a patient, a more accurate characterization is the recurrence of detectable cancer.

If prostate cancer comes back, well, it was never really gone. It was there, but undetectable. In my opinion and experience we should not burden ourselves with the hope and expectation of an absolute cure. We need to understand and accept that residual, undetectable cancer may remain after an apparently curative treatment, and we must be prepared for those undetected cells to divide, to spread, and to become detectable once again.

There are many realities with prostate cancer. A man facing unfavorable screening might in fact not have cancer, as Andrew came to find out. At the opposite extreme, a man's cancer can go undetected until it is too late for curative treatment and only palliative care (relief from symptoms) is warranted, as Joe faced. Or the cancer may not warrant treatment for a variety of reasons, such as apparent low risk, so medically supervised monitoring is the strategy, as with Peter. On the other hand, the cancer threat could warrant treatment despite serious and permanent side effects. For George, he did not know how serious his cancer threat was. He just knew he had cancer and wanted it gone, despite the side effects.

To simplify the process and to frame the cancer's aggressiveness, I sought to answer this question: Is it a sheep or a wolf? Building on the concept, as to where all the cancer might be, I thought of the prostate gland as "the barn," the area surrounding the gland as the "barnyard," and the lymph nodes as "checkpoints." I saw the blood vessels as the "highway" to distant organ metastasis, incurable disease.

With nonaggressive "sheep" cancer in the barn, there would be time to consider and decide upon a treatment method. If they were in the barnyard, one would face an increasing threat. Sheep at the checkpoints present an even greater challenge. If the sheep were out onto the highway, or if the cancer were a dangerously aggressive "wolf," even in the barn, I don't see how there could be calm. Using these analogies made it easier for me to comprehend the diagnostic and treatment challenges.

As to whether I had sheep or wolves, fortunately I had sheep. Mean ones though, as they got out of the barn and spread to several checkpoints. As to the question of whether we got all the cancer, I came to learn this cannot be completely answered.

My Cancer Story's Genesis Began in England

Through several turns of fate, and as my children were independent adults, I came to be living in England. I owned a small software company that had acquired another small business in England. After several years of attempting to lead that office from Austin, it was necessary to take full-management control. To do that I obtained a UK Tier 1 Entrepreneur visa and established myself in an apartment, outside of London.

More than an apartment, my residence was the bottom floor of the Waltons bed-and-breakfast, a classic Victorian home on Rose Hill in the wonderful, historic market town of Dorking, Surrey. The house is complete with lovely gardens and is a brief walk from the commerce of the High (main) Street area, including several favorite pubs where I spent evenings enjoying the company of friends and strangers alike. Other regulars of the Waltons and various neighbors on the hill became more than acquaintances. I am very fond of the proprietors Maggie and Richard, and they hosted my children and friends from the United States on numerous occasions. Most special were the

Christmas and New Year's holidays. We would gather regularly for food and drink, celebrating the festive season.

From the house, I hiked or ran directly into the Surrey hills, where there are seemingly endless trails to explore. Walks through the woods to distant pubs for Sunday supper were unique fun times. Outstanding hill country cycling routes started from the driveway. The Dorking and Mole Valley Athletics Club running group did track-style workouts in the winter months on the Rose Hill loop, directly in front of the house. This is where I met them. The opportunity to exercise right from my doorstep epitomized the kind of lifestyle that appealed to me.

One bit of Dorking history I am fond of is that William Mullins and his family traveled on the historic 1620 trip to America on the Pilgrim ship the *Mayflower*. Another contribution to history is the local residents' sacrifices to WWI and WWII. My walk from the Waltons to the office took me by the war memorial inscribed with the names of the Dorking men who gave their lives for my freedoms. Occasionally, I paused to read some of the names and say a solemn thank-you.

How the United Kingdom's and Europe's Approaches to Health Care Guided Me

Although my medical consultations were as a private, self-paying patient, the doctors I consulted with also practiced within the UK's National Health Service (NHS). My experiences were a welcomed and critical difference from my experiences in the United States. Simply put, I felt the approach to prostate screening and cancer treatment I experienced in Europe was superior to my experiences back home.

My experience began with a seemingly routine screening in London. However, the urologist examined my prostate in a far more thorough procedure than I had previously undergone. That examination identified a lesion (tumor) on my prostate gland. Without question, that lesion was missed in previous exams.

For further investigation the doctor recommended magnetic resonance imaging (MRI) of my prostate. That was the first time I'd heard of imaging of the prostate. That finding suggested cancer. A subsequent prostate biopsy confirmed cancer. Suddenly, the wonderful lifestyle I had established in Dorking was at risk.

Despite my US urologist's recommendation for immediate surgery, I returned to London, and I am glad I did. There I learned of diagnostic methods and treatment options I had not heard of back home. It took nine months of patient-style research and many medical consultations before I made my treatment decision. My choice was surgery, a prostatectomy, the very treatment method I'd tried to avoid. I had that done at home, in Austin, Texas. Eleven months later I began radiotherapy in an attempt to kill the small amount of remaining cancer. When that proved unsuccessful I returned to Europe for advanced imaging, a nanoparticle MRI, in the Netherlands. Five lymph nodes were identified as suspect for cancer. With more research and consultations with doctors in the USA and Europe, I traveled to Belgium for surgery to remove my pelvic lymph nodes; known as *salvage lymphadenectomy*.

Believing that cancer is a lifelong journey and accepting that there is no absolute assurance of a cure, following that surgery I began hormone therapy, antiandrogen (a testosterone blocker) drug treatment as a precautionary strategy. The specific drug I choose, bicalutamide, is from the UK. My surgeon in Belgium recommended it. Although known to my American doctors, they recommended an "American" drug. I did my homework and based on my understanding, bicalutamide presented a lower risk for side effects. There was no objection to my preference.

Reflecting back, there are several practices in England that I wish were standard protocol in the USA. With each consultation I received a comprehensive letter from the doctor, including their findings and recommendations. I no longer had to rely on what I did or did not remember or got wrong. Also, instead of waiting for long periods in a soulless lobby, the doctors came out to greet me at the scheduled time. They introduced themselves by their first name and walked me to the consulting room. No nurse conducted a totally unnecessary check of my height, weight, body temperature, and blood pressure.

The most important practice that I got a glimpse of is the multidisciplinary team consultation approach. With this approach at least two specialists from each applicable discipline meet to discuss a case. They fully evaluate the thoroughness of the diagnosis, weighing the pros and cons of their respective treatment methods. The objective is to reach consensus as to which treatment method or methods would best serve each individual patient.

From my perspective, as the doctors do not lose income if they defer to another treatment, they are in a comfortable position to give their best advice; not biased by their potential to gain or lose financially. As a private self-paying patient, I did not fully experience that team approach, but I did see the open-mindedness of the doctors I met with, and I did not feel that they saw me as additional revenue potential. In fact, two doctors recommended that I should not use their treatment methods, thereby foregoing private patient income. How unbiased was that?

At the time of this book's publication in early 2019, my blood testing reflected no detectible cancer. Most gratefully, I have had no serious side effects from the four treatments I've undergone. I am very certain that without the medical consultations in London, the nanoparticle MRI in the Netherlands, and the surgery in Belgium, I would not be experiencing this most favorable outcome. Had I gone forward with the first recommendation for surgery, it might well be that all the cancer would have been removed, but I would have sacrificed my sexual nerves and possibly my continence. Furthermore, if that procedure had failed to get all the cancer, I might well have faced radiotherapy to the pelvic region, resulting in additional and permanent side effects, at the young age of sixty.

ONE

THE SCREENING CONUNDRUM

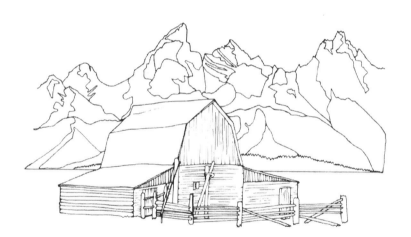

P rostate cancer is the leading cancer incidence in and the second leading cause of cancer death (behind lung cancer) in American men, as stated by the 2015 US Department of Health and Human Services Centers for Disease Control and Prevention.[6] Clearly, prostate cancer is a serious disease, yet there is no national screening program. Perhaps this is one reason so many men give this disease little concern.

According to the American Cancer Society's (ACS) February 2018 statistics, about one in nine men will be diagnosed with prostate cancer, and one man in forty-one will die of it. With an apparent emphasis, the ACS states that it develops mainly in older men. The ACS further identifies the average age of diagnosis at around sixty-six, and says that the majority of men with this disease do not die from it.[7] Are these statements offered to give men and society a calmness regarding this disease? To lower our concerns? I say they are examples of misinformation.

Logically, a national screening program would lower the average age of diagnosis, for clearly there are younger men with undetected prostate cancer. And if older men with other serious pressing health issues, coincidentally found to have a nonconcerning prostate cancer, were not included in the statistical group, the average reported age would go down further. Might then more men be concerned with and screen for this disease?

Does the ACS statement that most men with this disease do not die from it suggest that no man should be concerned?

Furthermore, does the statistic "one man in forty-one" dies from prostate cancer represent an acceptable loss of life?

If you have not yet started screening for prostate cancer, consider this: screening for colon cancer using colonoscopies is standard practice, and often free with health insurance at appropriate ages because of the financial advantages of detecting colon cancer early—yet more men die from prostate cancer than colon cancer.

Back in 1998, at the young and healthy age of forty-one, I began prostate cancer screenings as part of a wellness plan intended to ensure my continued good health well into retirement. My two children were young, and as a divorced father with sole parental and financial responsibility, it was imperative that I stay healthy. Given that prostate cancer and breast cancer are in my family now, I am concerned for my brother. Although he did have a screening, his doctor expressed little faith in it. It is my wish that he learns from me and will seek thorough screenings from a different doctor.

Had I not screened for prostate cancer, my disease would not have been identified in its earlier stage, leaving no scope for curative treatment. But it took the surprise finding of a lesion on my prostate gland for me to appreciate the perplexing mess that men are in regarding screening. All the misinformation on blood testing plus the limitations of physical examinations (which I learned about later) led me to become dangerously complacent. It remains a harsh reality that despite my early screening efforts, my cancer went needlessly undetected for too long.

Prostate-Specific Antigen (PSA) Blood Test

Introduced in the 1980s, this test measures the level of a specific antigen in a man's blood, a protein that is made only by the prostate gland. The results are reported as the concentration of the antigen in nanograms (ng), one billionth of a gram, per milliliter (mL) of blood. The amount of this antigen detected in the blood is an indicator of a man's age and the health of his prostate.

Because the test is an indicator and not an absolute, definitive result, there is no established norm. What men have to work with is a reference range that may or may not indicate prostate cancer. One established guideline is 0.00–4.00 ng/mL, as my own laboratory reports reflected. Additionally, my reports noted *"In healthy males without prostatectomy, the reference interval is 4.00 ng/mL or less."*

It is commonly written that an elevated PSA level remains the single best indicator of prostate cancer,[8] and a level above 3 or 4 ng/mL warrants additional evaluation.[9] One criticism of this screening technique, however, is that most men with an elevated PSA do not have prostate cancer. Another is that prostate cancer may well be present even with a low PSA. Then there is the claim that many cancers detected by this method are not life threatening. Shouldn't the focus be on finding life-threatening cancer?

It seems the greatest criticism of this screening method is that elevated PSAs lead to unnecessary biopsies. Before overreacting further investigation with techniques such as imaging will provide additional information on the health of a man's prostate. Although no one wants an unnecessary biopsy procedure, as with elevated PSAs that are not from cancer, is it not also wonderful news when a man's prostate biopsy is negative?

That said, does a negative biopsy finding thereby make it unnecessary?

Digital Rectal Examination (DRE)

Approved for use in conjunction with the PSA test in the early 1990s, this physical examination is another check of the overall health of the prostate gland. Being digital, I thought it would be done with an instrument. Initially my exams were performed by GPs. Later they were done by urologists. They all used the same examination procedure. You are asked to lower your pants and underwear, and then bend over the exam table. The doctor gently inserts a gloved and lubricated finger into the rectum to examine the gland. Although a bit uncomfortable, they are painless and quick. The finding we want is an "all clear," meaning that no tumor or hardness was felt by the doctor.

A major criticism of DREs is that they can miss early-stage prostate cancer, as in my case. Another is that all too often when they do identify cancer, it is in a later, less treatable stage.[10] It was possibly too late for me when I came to understand that an all clear can be a false indicator, proving a negative is not always a negative.

In other words, the all clear does not mean a man does not have prostate cancer. What it indicates is that the doctor did not *feel* hardness, the tumor, the cancer that could be present. Each man being examined by this method must fully understand these limitations of the DRE. In chapter 3, the section "Upheaval," I will describe in detail how a more thorough DRE identified the tumor on my prostate gland.

To Screen or Not to Screen?

Looking back, had I known a few years earlier what I know now, my cancer would have been diagnosed and treated before it had spread as far as it did. As patients we have a critical role in our health care decisions. With easy access to considerable medical information, we have the opportunity to be patient detectives, patient scientists, and thereby capable self-advocates. We must look beyond what can be a murky suspicion from PSA and DRE screening, indicating that cancer may or may not be present.

Until 2017 the United States Preventative Services Task Force (USPSTF) recommended against routine prostate cancer screening for average-risk men of all ages. On May 8, 2018, they published a final new recommendation statement:

> *Based on a review of the current evidence, the Task Force recommends that men aged 55 to 69 years make an individual decision about whether to be screened after a conversation with their clinician about the potential benefits and harms. For men 70 years and older, the potential benefits do not outweigh the expected harms, and these men should not be routinely screened for prostate cancer.*[11]

Well, the *"potential benefit"* has unquestionably extended my life, and perhaps saved me from death due to prostate cancer. As for the potential harms, I believe they are the result of false conclusions and wrong judgments by the medical industry, its practitioners and, as in my case, the patient as well. For nowhere in medical journals or even in a single article could I find scientific evidence citing faults of PSA measurements, suggesting that they can be numerically inaccurate, such as thermometers or weight scales might be. And if during a DRE the doctor cannot feel a tumor that may in fact be there, the doctor's report is accurate—since the doctor did not feel it.

The United States is not alone in its position toward this aspect of men's health care. For example, neither the Canadian[12] nor the UK[13] health systems offer routine prostate cancer screening, except for men in high-risk categories. Yet, like the screening contradiction in the US, colon cancer screening with colonoscopies are routinely offered at age fifty-five to all residents in England.

Is the apparent government logic that because historically the PSA test and the DRE have led to "unnecessary biopsies and unnecessary treatments" men should not do routine screenings? And are these public policies based on the idea that the benefits of offering universal screening are outweighed by the cost to the overall population? In my opinion that thinking is certainly crazy logic for a disease as common as prostate cancer.

Why not let us put the focus on very thorough diagnostic techniques and finding cancer in its earlier stage, giving men the opportunity for successful treatment? And let us relish the fact that most men with seemingly unfavorable screening results do not have prostate cancer, rather than finding harm in those with favorable outcomes.

Imaging: The Key to More Thorough Evaluation

Why isn't imaging a standard screening method for prostate cancer detection? After all, mammograms are a standard screening method for breast cancer and colonoscopies are the standard screening procedure for colon cancer. And why did I have to go to Europe for the opportunity to obtain the most advanced imaging technology available?

Is it that cost/benefit ratios are considered too high given that the average age for diagnosis is considered old and that the death rate, regardless of age, is simply an acceptable loss of life? All this makes me wonder what we define as best medical practice for prostate cancer detection and treatment.

Even basic imaging can eliminate the so-called unnecessary biopsy procedure. And with increased frequency imaging is being used to target biopsy procedures to the more concerning area of a tumor, thereby reducing the number of needle samples, infections and prolonged bleeding.[14]

With advancements in diagnostic methodologies prostate cancer should no longer go undetected until it is too late for successful treatment. Imaging methodologies include MRI scans, positron emission tomography (PET) scans and computed tomography (CT). The ones I became familiar with are choline PET CT, fluciclovine PET CT and prostate-specific membrane antigen (PSMA) PET CT. After a prostatectomy and radiotherapy failed to get all my cancer I traveled to the Netherlands for the most advanced imaging available at that time, a PSMA PET CT combined with a nanoparticle MRI.

Might imaging have helped our friends in the prologue? For Andrew, perhaps his surgery could have been avoided. For George, imaging might have provided a sense of reassurance and led to additional investigations, delaying his rush to surgery based mainly on fear. For Joe, might imaging have shown his cancer had metastasized, forgoing the need for a surgery that was abandoned? And for Peter, might imaging and additional investigations provided him with a better understanding of his risk level?

While camping in the Grand Teton National Park, Wyoming, in September 2016, I came across a medical conference being held at the park's Jackson Lake Lodge; the World Molecular Imaging Society's "Imaging in 2020—The Future of Precision Medicine: Molecular Imaging for Diagnosis and Surgery/ Therapy." Well, I had to have a look, so I invited myself into the opening night's welcoming reception. My presence was warmly received, and I had the opportunity for a few quick chats with renowned doctors and scientists. It turns out there were several presentations on the advances that are being made in the early detection of prostate cancer. Clearly, the ambition of the doctors and scientists who attended the conference is to develop advanced imaging technologies that will significantly benefit men and women worldwide. Although it may be years before every local medical practice realizes these advances, it seems logical to me that every doctor should use what imaging technologies they have, and advise patients of what may be available elsewhere.

TWO

HOW SCREENING FAILED ME

1998-2014

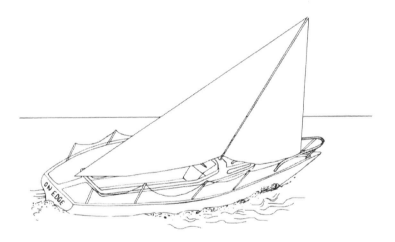

My father was a capable sailor. He was raised near the San Francisco Bay and built his own boats in his youth. He introduced me to sailing and I was hooked. My boat is a 1970s sloop named *On Edge*. I joke that it's named for my personality, but it's because of how she heels over on the gunwale, the edge, in good winds. It's great fun. I often feel on edge with screening, but that is never fun.

From 1998 through 2004 my PSA blood levels were within the standard range guideline 0.00–4.00 ng/mL and my DRE physical examinations were always clear. With such favorable results it was natural and logical for me to take comfort, to have no worries, no fears.

Then unexpectedly in September 2004, at the age of forty-seven, my annual screening came back with a high and frightening result, 20.4 ng/mL, suggesting serious cancer. I was immediately referred to a specialist. Despite my DRE being clear I was told to prepare for the worst and a prostate biopsy was urgently scheduled.

Waiting for the procedure and the subsequent report was an anxious time. As things happened so quickly I kept the cancer scare to myself. My daughter, Shannon, and my son, Matthew, weighed heavily on my mind. What would their futures be without me, without a loving, caring parent in their lives? When the doctor called with the results, all was put right. The biopsy finding was benign. No cancer. My elevated PSA was a false indicator—but why? We scheduled a follow-up appointment and I began researching for answers.

It turns out that in addition to cancer, antigen levels in the blood can be increased by prostate gland infections, sexual activity, and bicycle riding. So if one has an infection, or participates in sexual activity or bicycling in the days before the blood sample is taken, a rise in PSA may occur. Well, I was an avid bicyclist and my girlfriend was sexually adventurous; she enjoyed stimulating me with prostate massages. In the follow-up visit I shared my pre-blood test activities with the doctor and without hesitation he felt they were the cause of that frightening spike.

As reflected in graph 1, not doing those activities in the days preceding testing immediately lowered my PSA levels and they held within the standard range guideline for the next five years.

Graph 1: PSA Spike and Fall

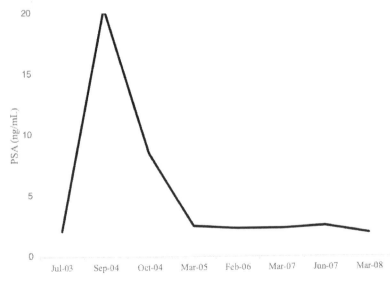

Note: Laboratory standard range guideline 0.00–4.00 ng/mL

In the years that followed, DRE physical examinations reflected that my prostate gland was enlarging, which is considered natural with aging. The symptoms can be very annoying, including multiple and urgent nightly bathroom runs, trouble starting urination, leaking, and dribbling. They can creep into the daytime hours as well. Fortunately, I did not face unmanageable issues or health concerns with my enlarged gland, so I declined medication to treat the condition. For men that are not as fortunate as I was, the medicine and physical treatment options can be complicated. From other men I know that face severe symptoms with an enlarged prostate, I learned they must choose between relief and side effects of treatment. As with prostate cancer, I think it is important for men to carefully research all the available information regarding treatment of an enlarged prostate, and to seek multiple diagnosis and treatment opinions.

In 2009 my PSA rose above 3.0 ng/mL but my urologist and I brushed that off because it was below the 4.0 guideline threshold, my DRE was all clear and I had entered my fifties, when levels are expected to naturally rise. In hindsight, that was the beginning of my PSA complacency.

In 2010 my PSA rose above the guideline threshold to 4.2. That raised a biopsy discussion but as my DRE was clear I was reluctant to have one. That reluctance was based on misinformation—principally all the literature citing unnecessary biopsies and overtreatments brought on by elevated PSAs. Besides, my own negative experience six years prior with a benign biopsy, which some would have called unnecessary, seemed to validate that misinformation. Falsely confident in my screening results and as I was in continued excellent health, I waited over two years for my next screening.

25

In July 2012 my PSA rose to 4.8 ng/mL, but with no change in screening guidelines and my DRE all clear, my doctor and I concluded that a biopsy was not warranted. In May 2013 my PSA rose to 7.0, warranting a biopsy. To alleviate my hesitation, we retested. The result was an unexpected drop so we retested a second time. That presented a further drop so with no explanation for the two drops and with an all clear DRE my doctor and I agreed to forego the biopsy and screen in nine months.

In February 2014 my PSA jumped well above the 4.0 standard range threshold to 10.3 ng/mL. Because of the previous year's rise and fall we did a retest—a 50 percent drop. Although we still had no explanations for the drops our immediate concerns were alleviated, so we arbitrarily decided that the next test would before year's end. Besides, I was returning to England with business development opportunities on my mind, so I was not going to let another nebulous screening result get in my way. My plan was to get the next test in Dorking.

Having the blood test done in another country was very easy. I simply walked a short distance from my office down the Dorking High Street to the medical clinic with my US doctor's written order. Instead of having the clinic mail the report, I requested a pickup, as I enjoyed the walk. So easy, so casual. Well, as life can and does surprise us, that October 2014 blood test was a life-changing event. My walk back to the office was somber now that I knew I had to find a very good urologist. Soon.

With PSA screening it seems we focus solely on the test result, a singular number, and its apparent meaning. Retrospectively, graph 2 clearly shows that despite repeated drops there was a steady rising trend above the standard range. What we did not consider was that we were falsely dismissive of the very thing we were screening for. Cancer.

Graph 2: PSA Steadily Rising

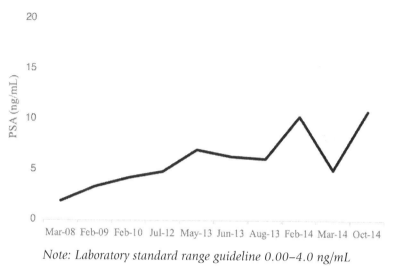

Note: *Laboratory standard range guideline 0.00–4.0 ng/mL*

The Perils of Screening Complacency

There is considerable information in the public domain regarding the pros and cons of PSA screening. The cons seem to be based on the reality that despite PSA screening being the best early indicator for prostate cancer, PSA can also be elevated when no cancer is present. So, the thinking is that elevated PSAs often lead to unwarranted anxieties and unneeded biopsies.

Every day now I regret how I let the sea of misinformation regarding prostate cancer screening override my purposeful intentions that I so responsibly initiated at forty-one. After a false alarm and having taken in all the misinformation I slipped into a state of screening complacency. As my PSA began to rise and fluctuate I did not want to overreact. What I had failed to consider was that underreacting can lead to one's early and otherwise avoidable death, which may yet prove to be my fate.

Even though my first biopsy procedure felt invasive and for months afterward there was blood in my urine, in retrospect I do not view it as unnecessary. And men, if we think it through, a prostate biopsy is similar enough to a colonoscopy, except that folks in the USA do use anesthesia Interestingly, I have been told that in Europe doctors generally do colonoscopies without anesthesia And gents, compared to childbirth, do we really have anything to whine about with prostate biopsies?

Regarding DREs, why do we so faithfully accept the "all clear" finding when it is widely published that DREs miss early-stage cancers? I relied heavily on my all clear findings—but to my own peril.

Today I view all the critical talk regarding screening and the claims of unnecessary prostate biopsies as systemic misinformation. Looking back, I now wonder when my cancer had started to develop. It seems logical based on timelines and the spread of my cancer that it was before my own PSA reached the 4.0 ng/mL threshold.

And oh, how I wish I had thought to graph my results during my years of screening. More importantly, how I wish I had known earlier about the role of MRIs for prostate cancer investigation and better targeted biopsies.

THREE

OH BOLLOCKS!
PROSTATE CANCER

October 2014–March 2015

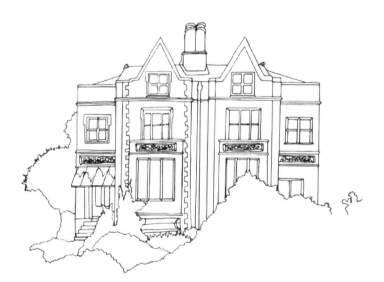

n England, saying "oh bollocks" is akin to and yet a much more acceptable way of saying "oh s—!"

The English autumn weather was excellent for cycling and hiking which accentuated how happy I was with my circumstances and lifestyle in Dorking. Extra special and most exciting for me was that Shannon, then twenty-eight, and Matthew, twenty-six, were coming over for a winter holiday. Shannon was making her third visit. It was Matthew's first. We had not shared an extended family trip together for a number of years, as they had developed their own lives. In addition to planning the holiday details, I needed to see a urologist.

Upheaval

Dr. Richard Brown, a GP and medical business consultant, was a regular guest at the Waltons bed-and-breakfast, which I wrote of in the introduction. Having two Richard Browns in the house often confused new guests, but the regulars knew we had the pleasure of both Richard Brown, husband to proprietor Maggie Walton, and Dr. Brown the guest.

Dr. Brown and I become friends over stimulating and provocative breakfast conversations, as well as occasional pints at Dorking's The Old House, a traditional English pub with ceiling beams older than my country. The newest proprietors, Joel and Aggie, renovated the pub and made something quite special, including beach hut–style patio seating and a secret door leading to a Narnia-like library; perhaps one day I might have a book signing there.

One morning at breakfast with Dr. Brown, I brought up the sensitive and personal discussion of prostate issues. Specifically, I asked him to recommend a urologist with leading-edge skills in diagnostic techniques who would be open to a patient who was knowledgeable (or so I thought) and in control of their health care. Richard made inquiries with his colleagues and referred me to Mr. Sarb Sandhu, consultant urologist, New Victoria Hospital, London. (In a quaint British tradition, surgeons use the title Mr. to reflect their historical status as meat butchers.)

That routine appointment was scheduled for a Sunday in early December. Turns out, doctors in the United Kingdom who also work under the public health service often schedule their private practice patient appointments during evenings and on weekends.

Mr. Sandhu greeted me in the waiting area and introduced himself as Sarb. He took me to his consultation room and opened a friendly easy discussion. We reviewed my entire prostate screening history. With the current PSA spike, Mr. Sandhu recommended a DRE, explaining it would be different than my previous exams. Instead of lowering my drawers and bending over the exam table as with all previous exams, I removed the clothes below my waist and lay on the table. As he examined me I was instructed to extend and contract my legs so he could adequately feel the whole of the gland.

As a result of that very thorough examination, Mr. Sandhu felt a lesion on my prostate. With care and patience, he explained that it was a small tumor and he assured me that I had no cause for immediate alarm.

To further investigate my prostate health, he recommended an MRI, explaining that they were common in private practice as an additional screening tool. If an abnormality were seen, the images would be used to target biopsies to precise areas of tumors, thereby limiting the number of possible locations from which samples needed to be taken. As the holidays and the arrival of Shannon and Matthew were weeks away, we scheduled the MRI for January. Prior to their arrival, I decided I would not share my medical concerns with them, as I had insufficient information and my health was not in imminent danger.

In addition to a week based in Dorking, we had trips planned to Rome and Venice. One characteristic of our travels is that we go as hard and long as we can each day. This began upon their arrival. Despite having flown overnight from Austin to London Heathrow, we grabbed their bags and headed straight off to tour nearby Hampton Court, one of King Henry VIII's palaces. Later that evening and back at the Waltons, we dined with Maggie and Richard.

Throughout the week favorable weather allowed for walks in the Surrey hills and quick trips to London. A favorite festivity was Hyde Park's Winter Wonderland, with fun rides, tasty foods and mulled wines, singing and dancing. Several evenings we visited with friends while pub hopping. All our activities captured the Christmas spirit, yet it was not always easy balancing the holiday festivities while having the tumor on my mind.

When our week in England wrapped up, we flew to Rome. In addition to all the exciting things to see and do, the look on Matthew's face as we walked around the Colosseum made everything seem right. On Christmas Day we traveled by train to Venice. Of all the sights to see, Shannon and I were especially looking forward to art galleries and museums, although

33

we were hesitant about Matthew's interest. To our surprise, Matthew really enjoyed the galleries, and pointed out details in paintings we simply missed. After three nights in Venice we returned to England.

Our family holiday was amazing, with the highlight being the wonderful respect and hospitality Matthew received in Italy. Words cannot describe how kind, warm, and generous the Italians were in respect of his severe physical disabilities. Matthew was born with multiple birth defects. He has no arms, and only a couple of digits extend from each shoulder. He also deals with very poor hearing, requiring a hearing aid, and kidney disease, but despite his challenges Matthew gets on with things.

After saying goodbye to Shannon and Matthew at Heathrow Airport for their return to Austin my thoughts shifted to the upcoming MRI. As things can happen the hospital had a scheduling conflict so the January appointment was rescheduled for February. Days before that appointment I was knocked off my feet with a serious English winter cold (often called "man flu" there), resulting in another cancellation.

With an upcoming trip to warmer, drier, sunnier Texas I emailed my urologist in Austin advising him of the lesion and inquired as to the possibility of an MRI. To my surprise he supported the idea and one was scheduled. It struck me how easy that was, even though no American doctor had mentioned prostate MRIs, nor had I learned of them in my early readings. Obviously available, but as I experienced, not often utilized or discussed.

MRI Indicates Significant Disease

I studied up on the procedure and was prepared for an uncomfortable exam. Various documents cited that standard practices used intravenous therapy (IVs) for contrast injections and an endorectal coil to enhance the images. The coil is a metallic tube that is inserted through the rectum. While I did get an IV needle placed in my arm, I was spared the endorectal coil. Advancements in the facility's MRI procedure no longer required the wire coil for imaging enhancements, which was a relief.

The procedure took about thirty minutes. My role was to lie on the medical table that took me into the imaging chamber. Despite the machine being noisy and confining, the circumstances were manageable. The contrast injection fluid was administered toward the later stage of the imaging process. Having fluids pumped into my arm was an unusual sensation.

The next day I saw my hometown GP for a general physical and he accessed my report online. The small tumor was located at the left bottom of the prostate gland, in a narrow area known as the apex. The unexpected and frightening information was that significant disease was likely present. Although I had been very reluctant to have another biopsy the findings convinced me one was necessary. I called my urologist's office and was able to schedule a biopsy straightaway. Suddenly that trip home was not going to be the fun in the sun I had planned so with the biopsy scheduled I postponed my return to London.

As my knowledge progressed, I came to understand it was the tumor's close proximity to the urethra that would call into question whether treatment was even possible without serious risk to my continence. Of even greater concern was that this opening is essentially an open barn door for the cancer cells to spread through. Without the MRI we would not have had this knowledge. Why any doctor or patient would go forward with treatment without the crucial details available from an MRI is inconceivable to me.

Biopsy

Radiological tests are excellent diagnostic tools, but they are not used to give an absolute diagnosis of cancer because a tissue sample for microscopic examination is not collected. To obtain tissue samples a prostate gland biopsy is performed and having had two I can say they are unpleasant.

A spring-loaded trigger-activated needle is used for the procedure. The device is not small and it is a painful squeeze as it is inserted into the rectum. When "fired" it makes a disturbing noise and feels like a stinging bite. Typically, twelve or more tissue samples are taken to ensure adequate sampling of the gland. This involves the doctor rotating and repositioning the device, an unpleasant experience. Ouch!

Lying on the procedure table with knowledge about the use of MRIs to better target the biopsy needle, I attempted to negotiate (reduce) the number of samples that would be taken from my prostate. After a brief give-and-take the doctor and I agreed to six core tissue samples, less than half the number taken in my biopsy years earlier.

Immediately the procedure was uncomfortably painful as the doctor had difficulty inserting the biopsy needle into my rectum. He suggested we reschedule the procedure and do it under full anesthesia but that alternative was not compelling so I asked for a few moments to relax. Somehow that worked and the procedure continued without further difficulty. In sharp contrast to my first biopsy I was spared the months of blood in my urine that I had experienced. I attribute that little success to the lesser number of tissue samples taken.

Pathology Report

Pathology: *The science of the causes and effects of disease, especially the branch of medicine that deals with laboratory examination of samples of body tissue for diagnostic or forensic purposes.* [15]

When I scheduled the biopsy appointment I requested that a copy of the pathology report be sent directly to me via email and confirmed that at check in. Despite the second procedure being less traumatic the week-long wait for the pathology report was as frightening as the first. While waiting I did my homework and was reasonably well-versed on the applicable medical terms.

The report arrived as an email attachment and when I opened it the verdict was right in my face. Big, capitalized bolded red text. CARCINOMA. For me that was a shocking way to present the finding and it took effort to work through that before reading the entirety of the report.

It did not take long for me to grasp the big picture. I had an established cancer with growth into nerve tissue. The presence of precancerous cells indicated the cancer had begun years earlier. I focused on the Gleason score—a prostate cancer grading system developed by pathologist Dr. Donald F. Gleason in the 1960s (which seems long ago). It describes the tumor cells' degree of abnormality as compared to healthy cells. The score would help identify whether my cancer was a sheep or wolf. This is how I understood it.

Gleason's system identifies five cellular patterns that indicate how far a cell has deviated from normal, denoted as patterns 1–5. Patterns 1 and 2 are considered benign; not cancer. Patterns 3, 4, and 5 reflect a worsening progression toward cancer, respectively. To obtain a score, the two most common patterns found within the cells taken by the tumor biopsy are added together. A combined score of 5 or below is regarded as a benign noncancerous finding. The lowest combined Gleason score that indicates cancer is 6. The higher scores of 8, 9, and 10 are considered high-grade, dangerous cancers. Wolves!

For example, if the most common cell pattern is 2 and the next most common pattern is 1, the score would be 2 + 1 = 3; not cancer. If the most common pattern is 3 and the next is 4, the score would be 3 + 4 = 7; cancer. Conversely, if there is more pattern 4 than pattern 3, the score is expressed as 4 + 3, a greater threat.

My Gleason score from that pathology report was 3 + 3 = 6. As a score of 5 is not cancer, and the worst possible score is a 10, I did not panic. But as with PSA, Gleason scores are subject to different interpretations, so there is justification for patient confusion and worry. Specifically, I read in several publications that a Gleason score 6 is often considered low-grade and not likely to rapidly grow and spread.[16] That information raised immediate questions—does my Gleason 6 warrant treatment, and if so, how and when?

Recommendation for Immediate Surgery

Having studied my pathology report I was ready to meet with my urologist in Austin. After years of screening we had established a good doctor-patient relationship. Immediately I brought up the report's presentation of cancer in red capital letters. He explained that was to ensure that the finding was not overlooked or missed completely. I expressed my shock and dismay with the presentation. Months later I received two additional independent pathology reports, and neither presented *carcinoma* in big, capitalized, bold, or red text.

We discussed how serious he thought the cancer was. The apparent good news was that the cancer posed no immediate threat and the doctor estimated it might take ten years for the onset of symptoms of distant organ metastasis. So, if I had ten years until symptoms and say another year until death from the disease, unless of course something else had killed me, I would be seventy. Would that be death by an old man's disease? And thereby an acceptable statistical loss of life to the system?

Despite no immediate threat and the ten-year estimate to symptoms, my doctor recommended surgery, a radical prostatectomy, the very next week. Perplexed, I focused on the Gleason 6 score, and cited multiple medical sources questioning whether the score warranted immediate treatment. He explained that in his opinion the tumor was cancerous, that treatment was needed, and he maintained his recommendation for immediate surgery. Looking back, it disturbs me that the doctor expressed no interest in assessing how aggressive my cancer was. Nor did he express concern as to whether my cancer had spread.

The discussion moved to the risks associated with surgery; he felt the procedure would not leave me with urinary incontinence, as it had in the case of George from our prologue. I asked how many lymph nodes would be removed and if the sexual nerves would be spared. His answer was that it was not the time to be conservative—that *we* wanted to do all that could be done to get *"all the cancer."* I tried to negotiate but that went nowhere. He took the conversation back to surgery.

Whoa, hold the horses, put on the brakes! Respected medical journals raise questions as to whether Gleason 6 cancer should be treated, let alone even considered cancer. Adding to my concerns were the widely publicized articles and books regarding overtreatments and the life-changing side effects that can come with treatment. With so much to consider I said no to immediate surgery.

Confused, and uncertain where to put my trust, I decided to return to London and scheduled an appointment with Mr. Sandhu, the doctor who detected my tumor and recommended that I have an MRI. In preparation for the consultation I had my MRI and pathology reports sent to him.

FOUR

MEDICAL AND TREATMENT CONSULTATIONS IN THE UNITED KINGDOM

April-July 2015

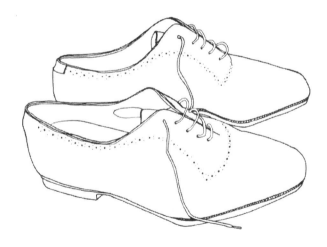

P atient-driven health care must be one of the most self-demanding processes a person can work through. In one's efforts and struggles not to be seen through the filters of statistics and probabilities, one must see themselves as an individual human who has the right to a considered-and-balanced diagnosis and treatment decision, in what is their entirely personal experience with cancer.

With my planned return to London I shifted my energies from business development to researching prostate cancer. Quickly I realized the task in front of me was large, even larger than I could have imagined. Although the internet was a key resource, it was also a nightmare. And Doctor Google was not nearly as helpful as one might expect. Plus, I faced financial expenditures I had not planned for; medical consultations, investigative tests and treatment methods that would not be covered by the private health insurance I had maintained back home.

Although I am not wealthy, I had a solid financial base to support my efforts. From my parents I learned the basics of personal financial management, including saving for rainy days. In a high school economics course I was introduced to financial wealth building. Based on those teachings I strived to live well within my means and to be debt-free. For me this means having a smaller home, modest vehicles and toys. It was those very practices that provided me the funds to handle all the rainy days of medical expenses.

A Different Perspective

For my consultation with Mr. Sandhu I knew I wanted someone with me to confirm what I heard, so I asked Annie, my first friend in Dorking to accompany me. Mr. Sandhu warmly welcomed us into his consultation office, and we got right to it. He accepted the MRI and biopsy findings of cancer and believed treatment was likely warranted, given my younger age and otherwise excellent health. However, he disagreed with the recommendation for immediate surgery and based his opinions on multiple factors. The MRI and pathology findings clearly indicated a smaller, lower-risk cancer that most likely had not yet metastasized to distant organs. He then explained that with lower-grade localized prostate cancer there is time to determine the risks and make a treatment decision. Now that was surely a different perspective than the recommendation for immediate surgery, and a lot to take in. I was grateful that Annie was with me.

44

One option for managing prostate cancer is watchful waiting, or active surveillance, as our friend Peter in the prologue was doing. My understanding of active surveillance is that even though a man has prostate cancer, no treatment is planned. Mr. Sandhu and I discussed and promptly dismissed this approach. So, if I needed treatment, but not immediately, what were my options?

Mr. Sandhu provided information on two alternative non-surgical-treatment methods, the CyberKnife radiosurgery system and HIFU, which utilizes high-frequency ultrasound energy to heat and destroy cancer cells. I expressed my concerns regarding radiation but Mr. Sandhu very reassuringly explained some of the advances in treatment techniques. Intrigued with both methods, Mr. Sandhu offered to make referrals and arranged for appointments on my behalf. While awaiting the appointments I booked a last-minute getaway ski trip with the Ski Club of Great Britain. It was on that trip that I met Dr. Carole Wyatt who graciously wrote the foreword for this book.

Tired each day from skiing I used the restful evenings to read up on radiotherapy. Alternatively called radiation therapy, or abbreviated as RT, it is a primary and secondary cancer treatment intended to kill or control the spread of malignant cells. I learned there are two principal methods: external-beam radiation and internal radiation (brachytherapy) utilizing radiation seeds or pellets. At that point in my journey I was considering radiotherapy for primary treatment; a year-and-a-half later I used it for secondary treatment.

The CyberKnife Robotic Radiosurgery System

The name sounded leading edge: clean and precise. Simply described, CyberKnife robotic radiosurgery is very targeted external-beam radiation. The nonsurgical aspect appealed to me, but there were risks. I understood that over time the onset of urinary incontinence and sexual dysfunction were possible. I appreciated that because the treatment would be focal (localized), the risks for tissue damage to the bowel and pelvic region lymphatic system were reduced.

Refreshed from my ski holiday and reasonably informed on the uses of radiotherapy, I was ready for the consultation with Dr. van As, one of England's top oncologists and a CyberKnife specialist. The Royal Marsden hospital where he practiced is of the stature of the Mayo Clinic, MD Anderson, and Johns Hopkins cancer treatment centers in the US.

In support, Annie joined me for this consultation. Dr. van As had my MRI images displayed on his monitor and written

45

medical reports in hand. Like Mr. Sandhu, he believed my cancer was diagnosed at an earlier stage and that time was on my side. That was reassuring. But then he raised numerous concerns that drove my continued research.

Based on the MRI Dr. van As was hesitant to accept the pathology finding of Gleason 3 + 3, which they did not always treat. He thought the finding might be under-scored on the Gleason scale and recommended a second pathology review, to be done by the Royal Marsden. If one or both of my Gleason 3 scores were actually a 4, that would indicate a more serious cancer. I agreed to the second review and arranged for my biopsy slides to be sent from Austin.

Again referring to the MRI, Dr. van As emphasized concerns about the tumor's location, which was close to the apex and the sphincter muscles. He felt that location would not allow for sufficient treatment margins. I came to understand that treatment margins are the untreated tissues between the tumor and the other surrounding tissues and organs. The objective is to leave sufficient margins so as to not damage the surrounding tissues and organs, while being sure no cancer cells are left untreated. Specifically, he was concerned for damage to the sphincter muscles which would risk urinary incontinence. Lastly, he felt that if the radiation did not get all the cancer, residual scar tissue could interfere with follow-on surgery.

Dr. van As explained in conclusion that if treatment was warranted, as he suspected it was, he would recommend traditional surgery. His concerns validated my quest to fully understand the extent of the risk that the cancer posed to my lifestyle and my life. I left the consultation feeling privileged, thankful for the referral by Mr. Sandhu, and pleased with my decision to return to London.

High-Intensity Focused Ultrasound (HIFU)

My initial consultation was in early May 2015 with Professor Emberton, University College Hospital, London. Professor Emberton is a leading world authority on HIFU and imaging techniques for prostate cancer. I took the one-hour train ride from Dorking to London Victoria station, which I always enjoy, and met up with Carole. Although it had been a short time since we met on the ski trip, our friendship was growing and she'd offered to join me for the consultation. With time to spare we took a leisurely walk to the medical office and on arrival served ourselves tea. Before we finished our drinks Professor Emberton called for me. He welcomed us, introducing himself as Mark, and led us up the stairs to his consulting room.

After a brief exchange Professor Emberton directed the discussion to my MRI images. As did Dr. van As, he felt the images suggested areas of Gleason pattern 4. He explained that the images lacked certain details he was used to seeing, and that it seemed the biopsy needle had missed the most suspicious area of the tumor.

To investigate his concerns Professor Emberton recommended a second MRI, at a London facility he suggested. We would then consider another biopsy, possibly to be done under full anesthesia and with an entry point through the perineum. I had not heard of that approach. He explained that this method would provide direct access to the tumor area that needed to be sampled; it would be a true, targeted biopsy.

As Carole and I left the consultation I wanted to walk while I processed the opinion of Professor Emberton, which mirrored that of Dr. van As—that I likely faced a more serious cancer than was originally diagnosed. After a bit of window-shopping,

I took what I thought was a sensible diversion; I bought a fine pair of Barker England, whole-cut leather Oxford shoes.

Second Look at Surgery Back Home

As June 2015 approached, I prepared for a quick trip home for Shannon's second university graduation. Shannon's bachelor's degree is in neuroscience. Her second degree, following a change of heart (or head, as the case may be), qualified her as a doctor of pharmacy. Although it was reassuring to have a medical professional in the family, I was not yet ready to share my health situation with my children or my friends. I wanted a better understanding of my outlook and my plan.

Upon my return to Austin I met with my long-established urologist; the doctor who performed the biopsy three months earlier and recommended surgery straightaway, based on the Gleason 6 score. As always, he was friendly and open to my questions. I shared my consultations with Mr. Sandhu and Drs. van As and Emberton. We talked through their concerns for about the disparity between the MRI findings and the biopsy Gleason 6 score; specifically, their opinions that the MRI suggested a higher Gleason score. My urologist did not share their views and was quite clear in his opinion that there was no need for a second MRI or a second pathology review. In fact, he was quite critical of HIFU and emphasized that that procedure was experimental and not approved for use in the USA. I raised the argument that all proven procedures had to begin in an experimental phase, including the robotic surgery procedure he had recommended. But he was not moved, and stood firm on his recommendation for surgery straightaway. I again raised the questions of sexual-nerve sparing and the number of lymph nodes to be removed. As we were unable to come to a consensus, my position remained unchanged: no rush to surgery.

Although published information as to the exact date is confusing, HIFU was approved for use by the US Food and Drug Administration in late 2015.

A More Serious Cancer

As my quest for the best possible quality-of-life outcome continued, I returned to London for my appointment at Nuada Medical. Professor Emberton had recommended Nuada for good reasons and I took confidence in the proclamation posted at the facility: *"State-of-the-art precision diagnostics for nuanced care."* Although the mechanics of the procedure were essentially the same as the one done in Austin, the technology proved to be advanced.

In less than a week the MRI report arrived in the mail, as did the Royal Marsden pathology report which confirmed a more serious cancer with a higher Gleason score of 3 + 4 = 7. With those in hand I scheduled the follow-up consultation with Professor Emberton. Fellow Waltons' guest Dr. Richard Brown, who referred me to Mr. Sandhu, offered to accompany me as a friend.

Professor Emberton felt that the Nuada Medical MRI and the Royal Marsden pathology report provided sufficient information so that a targeted biopsy was no longer needed. To my disappointment he explained that HIFU would not be the best treatment method to clear my disease. In his consultation letter summarizing our discussions Professor Emberton wrote:

> *"The upgrading of the pathology (by Royal Marsden) was a surprise but concordant with the information gleaned*

*from [the first] MRI which suggested a higher-risk lesion.
The MRI done at Nuada suggests abutment to the upper
fibres of the sphincter but no direct sphincteric invasion.
This means that applying a margin to the lesion in focal
therapy will be compromised in terms of the amount [of
ultrasound energy]. This will result in a slightly increased
risk of residual cancer after treatment.*" Professor
Emberton further wrote, "*Surgery would be the best
approach to clear this disease as the margin is outside the
gland rather than inside the gland.*"

Those findings presented me a reasonable cause for concern;
that treatment, whichever method, might not clear all the cancer, because it was possibly already out of the barn. I realized
that I faced a difficult quality-of-life decision. Go forward with
treatment, risking life-changing side effects while not curing the
cancer, or accept the fate that I had an incurable disease that
would end my life in some ten-plus years. That was a tough way
to leave the medical consultation. As we left my friend Richard
knew I was shaken. Frankly speaking, I was more than shaken.
The additional information and greater awareness of my situation nearly brought me to my knees. I was grateful for Richard's
support and company.

Richard led the discussion as to where to go. Unwind in a
pub, eat dinner, or get the train back to Dorking? He then had a
great idea—as a player and a fan of tennis he suggested we take
a quick tube and bus ride over to Wimbledon and queue up
for a chance to watch the last tennis matches of the day. Upon
our arrival the scene was a bit disheartening; the queue was
long and moving slowly. Attendants suggested that our chance
of getting in was very low. Not wanting to be disappointed and

needing the diversion I convinced Richard we would stand and wait, relying on hope. Well, we did get in, and what fun we had watching several matches while enjoying a few pints of British ale.

On the train ride home I pondered whether I was grasping at straws or in a state of denial, but with careful thought I concluded I was neither grasping nor in denial. It was because of those consultations in London that I gained a better understanding of the risks the cancer posed to my health, lifestyle, and life. Unfortunately, the tumor's location precluded the CyberKnife and HIFU treatments. I had to keep looking.

As I had with my consultation with Dr. van As, I felt privileged to have the advice of Professor Emberton, and the referral by Mr. Sandhu.

A Most Privileged Consultation

My last medical consultation in England, albeit unofficial, was with Rose Hill neighbor Dr. John Wickham. A retired urologist and author, John had practiced in London at Saint Bartholomew's Hospital and the Institute of Urology. He was a pioneer of minimally invasive surgical techniques, often referred to as *keyhole surgery* and is considered one of the "godfathers" of robotic surgery.

John welcomed me into his home office and we discussed my cancer in great detail. He encouraged me to continue evaluating different treatment methods because he was concerned for the risks associated with surgery. John suggested I look into brachytherapy, which utilizes radioactive seeds (very small metal pellets) implanted into the prostate. The technique is generally used for men with early-stage, lower-risk cancers, and there are various combinations of external radiation and seeding that can be considered. Hearing this suggestion from none other than a godfather of robotic surgery was very compelling.

A personal note: On a return trip to Dorking in March 2017, I enjoyed tea with John and his wife Ann. Although not yet published, John shared a copy of his latest book with me, An Open and Shut Case: The Story of Keyhole or Minimally Invasive Surgery. *Before I could finish my book and share it with them, John Ewart Alfred Wickham died of heart disease on October 26, 2017.*

FIVE

ADDITIONAL CONSULTATIONS BACK HOME

July–December 2015

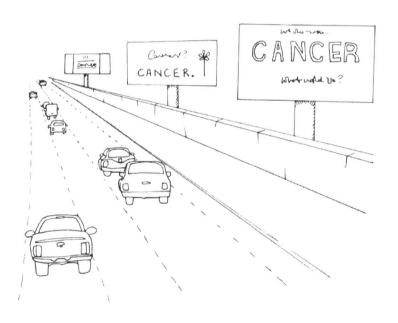

Whether or not I had treatment in England I could not remain a resident under my visa if I did not continue running my business. When I made the decision to close it down, I knew I would be returning home to Austin full-time. My long residency at the Waltons and the great English hospitality of Maggie and Richard was an amazing fun-filled experience. The day before my departure Maggie and Richard hosted a garden party. A wonderful way to say goodbye to my friends.

My residency in England officially ended in late July 2015. It was difficult to leave, and not only because of the cancer. I would surely miss Richard and Maggie and the neighbors of Rose Hill, the close friendships, and England and Europe as well.

The Texas hot I returned to was not the only heat I felt. I did a lot of thinking and reviewing of notes during the long flight home. I knew I needed treatment but remained hesitant of surgery, and was troubled by what I saw as different diagnoses of my cancer pathology. One a Gleason 6 score and the other a Gleason 7. That difference raised a serious question. How meek were my sheep? And I continued to ponder, what if the cancer had already spread into the barnyard, or worse, beyond? Could it be completely removed or killed by treatment, to never "come back"? If not, was ten years a good estimate to symptoms of distant organ metastasis? My quest for a good quality-of-life decision continued.

A Top Two Hospital

The University of Texas MD Anderson Cancer Center (MDA) is marketed as one of the original comprehensive cancer centers in the United States. It is rated as a top cancer care center in the "Best Hospitals" report published by *U.S. News & World Report*. As the MDA Houston facility was located near my daughter's new apartment, where she relocated following graduation, going there seemed like a no-brainer.

My intent was to explore the risk my cancer presented, and my treatment options, with a comprehensive medical team, a multidisciplinary approach, as is done in England. Scheduling the consultation was easy. What was unusual was that I was able to select the doctor I would first meet and that I was able to directly submit my medical records without the need for a referral. I appreciate that simplicity and direct relationship, as I experienced in England.

I have no doubt that wonderful work is done at MDA, and perhaps all their prospective patients are satisfied. That would be except me. Prior to meeting with the urologist I was called to a private business office where a professional representative went over financial matters and requested that I pay a large deposit. I questioned the deposit on the basis that I had medical insurance and my appointment was an initial consultation. It was explained to me that their policy was to collect the deposit. When I strongly objected the representative politely excused herself for a moment then returned with a much-reduced requirement. After a brief think I paid the new amount as I wanted to go forward with the consultation. The representative took me back to the waiting lobby.

Knowing what was next I calmed myself for the upcoming frustration. A nurse called my name for the weight, height, body temp and blood pressure dance. After that unnecessary check-the-box duet, I was taken to a patient room. An intern came in; that interaction was friendly and welcoming. We went over my history and data and he did a DRE, feeling my tumor. He left for a bit and then returned with the urologist. That conversation was strictly clinical and rushed. Simply put, he wanted to move forward with a radical prostatectomy. I wanted to begin a multidisciplinary consultation process with the excellent medical records I had provided. As that was not offered, I declined and that was the extent of the consultation. Although I left with no new information or insights, my parking fee was validated, and I received a prompt refund of the reduced deposit I had made.

In a strange way, that disappointing experience was reassuring in that I was confident and comfortable walking away from a leading cancer center. I had come to trust my own instincts in my health care decisions.

That evening during our warm-up jog Shannon and her fiancé Kyle asked about my day. Finally ready to share my health challenge with them I simply answered that I had been to MD Anderson Cancer Center, as a patient. We continued slow jogging with a comfortable honest discussion. Shannon, with her medical education, and Kyle, with his engineering education, were supportive of my process and approach. I was grateful for their love.

One-on-One with an Oncologist

As the scorching Texas August heat bore down on me, so did the pressures I was putting upon myself to find a cure. The pressures stemmed in part from all the advertising and marketing we face regarding cancer. Radio and TV commercials along with highway billboards promote the fight with cancer in many ways. One billboard in Austin promoting the CyberKnife method read *"WhenCancerComesBack.com—there's hope."* Since Dr. van As in London had recommended against the CyberKnife method for my circumstances, that advertisement was yet another source of misinformation.

To help me better understand my chances for a cure and my risk of the cancer coming back after treatment I wanted to meet with a medical oncologist, a specialist in the overall diagnosis and treatment of cancer. Unable to find one on my own, I asked my GP for a referral, which he quickly arranged.

My initial questions focused on the risk my cancer posed to my life. The doctor thought I had a lower-risk cancer that was likely still localized to the pelvic region. I accepted the possibility that the sheep were out of the barn, but not yet out onto the highway.

As the discussion progressed to treatment she realized my hesitancy and shared that if her husband were in my circumstances she would encourage him to have treatment, and sooner than later. That led to the question: was an absolute cure possible? Her straightforward answer was *no*; I could not be given that assurance. This is because although treatment can reduce prostate cancer to an undetectable level, today's medical science cannot absolutely determine if all cancer cells are successfully removed or killed by treatment.

Next, we discussed the possibility of my cancer coming back after treatment. That is when I came to appreciate that cancer does not "come back." I came to think of this like a splinter in one's finger. If you remove it all, it is all gone. Fail to remove it all and some remains.

An aspect of an unsuccessful treatment I came to appreciate was the elimination of the primary tumor, for that would slow the spread of any remaining cancer. I came to view this as a limited success, and most certainly not a failure.

Genomic Testing

After my consultation with the oncologist I sought out additional methods for determining the aggressiveness of my cancer. Carole and I were speaking more frequently and she was supporting my efforts to expand my knowledge and understanding. In one call she explained how as a breast cancer physician she relied upon genomic testing to indicate how aggressive a cancer was.

The test she used was the Oncotype DX assay from Genomic Health, an American company headquartered in Redwood City, California. I learned from their website that they had a specific test for prostate cancer. On the first phone call to the company I spoke with an informed representative and discussed whether the test was applicable to my particular circumstance. The representative felt it was but to have it done I needed to meet with a urologist familiar with its use and for my biopsy slides to be sent to their laboratory.

After several failed attempts with other doctors I went back to my principal urologist. He was familiar with the test and agreed to send my slides; the very slides from the biopsy he performed months earlier. Turns out the shipping of the slides took chasing on my part to get it done, so weeks were lost.

While I waited for the results from Genomic Health all my energies focused on Shannon and Kyle's upcoming September 2015 wedding in Seattle, Washington. They celebrated their marriage with close family and a few friends at the wedding venue site TreeHouse Point, near Seattle. We slept in very comfortable tree houses and enjoyed the beautiful forested grounds to ourselves for three nights. Matthew and I then joined Shannon and Kyle for kayaking fun off Orcas Island in Puget Sound and hiking in North Cascades National Park. We spent our last night together in Seattle.

Back in Austin I started planning for Carole's arrival from London. It was her first visit to the States and she received a wonderful Texas welcome, including the Austin City Limits Festival. Carole was excited to see the bands Hozier and Of Monsters and Men. We then embarked on an eight-hour drive to West Texas, heading to Big Bend National Park. Carole was overwhelmed by the wide-open space and skies of southwest Texas, which are quite unlike England. We enjoyed wonderful desert hikes and one evening were treated to an amazing desert lightning show above the Chisos Mountains. Our final destination before returning to Austin was Guadalupe Mountains National Park, where we enjoyed several climbs to the high peaks overlooking fall in the vast Chihuahuan Desert.

While driving home I received a call regarding my genomic test. The score would be reported as low-, intermediate-, or high-risk cancer. We listened calmly but intently to the technician as we rolled on down the highway. My Oncotype DX prostate score was low-intermediate risk. With that additional information I felt more comfortable with the paths I had chosen on my way to finding the most accurate diagnosis possible.

Now who would have thought this? That test, from a US company, was available in England to determine the aggression potential of various cancers, including of the prostate. To my surprise, it did not have US Food and Drug Administration approval for prostate cancer when I needed it in 2015. My private health insurance provider declined my claim and subsequent appeal, citing the test was experimental and unproven, and that they never anticipated approval. How wrong that statement was when two years later, in October 2017, Genomic Health announced final Medicare approval for prostate testing.[17] Such great news and progress for men seeking better ways to evaluate their prostate cancer risks and threats.

As October 2015 came to a close Carole returned to England and I continued on with research where, by chance, online advertisements caught my attention. One was for the Johns Hopkins medical second opinion program, the other for the Radiotherapy Clinics of Georgia.

Remote Medical Second Opinion Program

Johns Hopkins reputation speaks for itself. Additionally, I have a strong affinity for the university because Shannon earned her neurology degree from Hopkins. Having reviewed the second opinion program website I realized it was a different type of medical consultation; there would be no office visit, no physical exam, and no additional investigation. Instead it would be an analytical assessment based on medical records I provided. A detailed written medical review would be provided, including findings, recommendations, and answers to my submitted questions. I called upon my very supportive GP to submit my application and all applicable medical records. Submissions included the MRIs, biopsy pathology reports, and the Oncotype DX score.

The written report was the first I had received from an American doctor. It was comprehensive, covering each aspect of my diagnosis in considerable detail. It served as a benchmark against my recall and my own hastily written notes from other consultations and was a good substitute for a multidisciplinary approach. The report covered multiple treatment options and specifically recommended surgery. It emphasized that my continence should not be adversely affected—which was reassuring and consistent with most other opinions.

One statement addressed the questions raised by the doctors in England, based on the MRI findings, as to whether my cancer had spread. It stated that my cancer was *"likely already growing beyond the prostate."* It further stated that *"this does not mean it is not curable by local therapy"*—in other words, surgery or radiotherapy.

If my cancer had spread into the barnyard I realized treatment would require more than removal or killing of the gland. I gave thought to whether I had erred in saying no to the initial recommendation for a radical prostatectomy, and one that was not conservative in its reach. But I still maintain that if we do not know where all the cancer is, I am not willing to extend the reach of surgery to sexual nerves and many lymph nodes, which has been characterized as "lymph node chasing" and possibly overtreatment.

Brachytherapy Consultation

Recall in chapter 4, "A Privileged Consultation," that Dr. Wickham, a recognized pioneer of robotic surgery, suggested that I consider brachytherapy, radiotherapy utilizing radiation seeds or pellets, as an alternative to surgery.

What captured my interest in the Radiotherapy Clinics of Georgia advertisement was their focus on data. Intrigued, I made an online inquiry regarding their trademark procedure, "ProstRcision: The Proven Cure with NO Cutting." I received a prompt call from a patient representative for the clinic.

Following a useful conversation, I accepted the offer of an information package and found both the well-produced guidebook and DVD educational and encouraging.

To receive an evaluation for the likelihood of their treatment curing my cancer I forwarded my medical records to the clinic. To my surprise I received an evening call from Dr. Frank Critz, the founder of ProstRcision. We discussed details of my diagnosis. He then shared how they use data to calculate the likelihood of a successful treatment. Dr. Critz called twice more, and then sent a letter detailing the projected success rate with their procedure. It stated, *"If treated with ProstRcision, the fifteen-year chance of zero PSA (below 0.2 ng/mL) for Murray (Keith) Wadsworth is 89 percent."*

The projection was based on my cancer factors including my Gleason score, PSA, Oncotype DX score, and clinical stage. That was a promising outlook and a good alternative to full-on external-beam radiation or surgery.

A special note: Dr. Critz provided his consultation details in writing, personalized with his handwritten comments. To my pleasant surprise I was never charged for the review of my medical information, calls, letters, and analysis.

The Affordable Care Act (ACA)

In November 2015 I was pondering surgery at Johns Hopkins in Baltimore, Maryland or radiation treatment with Radiotherapy Clinics of Georgia in Atlanta, Georgia. With great shock to me my private insurance provider notified me by mail that they were canceling their (mine and tens of thousands of other individuals) preferred provider organization (PPO) health insurance plan in Texas, effective December 31, 2015. The reason given

63

for the cancellation was the additional costs and overly burdensome regulations brought upon by the ACA.

Suddenly, I found myself shopping for a new private health care insurance provider right in the middle of treatment decisions. To my further shock only a couple of companies offered plans to individuals in Central Texas and those had strict in-network coverage requirements and very limited out-of-network coverage. Simply put, I was losing my ability to choose my doctors, my preferred treatment methods and the facilities where I would receive them.

That unfortunate reality came to be recognized as a failed promise of the ACA. Although the ACA provided medical benefits to previously uninsured individuals, the costs and restrictions put upon those of us who always had insurance were very high. I found myself quite angry since all my adult life I had paid for private health insurance, either as an employee or as an employer. I never missed a single payment and never had a gap in coverage. Then suddenly my policy was cancelled and I could no longer purchase the type of coverage I'd had all my adult life. This happened because our elected representatives in Washington passed laws so that all could have more "affordable health care." Bollocks!

I did apply for a new plan and my application was accepted. With very limited or perhaps no out-of-network coverage I questioned the logic of self-funding the medical expenditures plus travel and housing costs that came with treatment at either Johns Hopkins or the Radiotherapy Clinics of Georgia. The pragmatic financial decision was to use doctors and medical facilities within my new insurance company's network, but that required finding new doctors. It seemed as if I was starting anew.

In another twist of fate, a year later my new insurance provider would cancel many thousands of individual coverage policies, including mine. For a second time I would be unexpectedly shopping for insurance right in the middle of my next round of treatment decisions. That second cancellation triggered a new concern: Would I have to shop for health insurance coverage every year?

Final Data Point

Notwithstanding convincing evidence that my cancer threat warranted treatment I found myself wanting a third independent pathology opinion. To help settle my concerns Carole contacted a former colleague and friend in England, a urologist, asking him which laboratory he would go to for a third pathology opinion. He regarded Bostwick Laboratories, Florida, as the "gold standard." So, my biopsy slides were sent to Bostwick Labs. Dr. Bostwick's findings concurred with those of the Royal Marsden: *the architectural features warrant a Gleason score of 3 + 4 = 7."* I was ready for treatment.

Decision Time

As 2015 came to its end my quest for a treatment decision that would best assure me of a continued high quality of life was completed. Recall that I was offered an appointment for surgery, a radical prostatectomy, the week following my cancer diagnosis, and that I said no. That was in March 2015. By December I had in hand two MRIs; three biopsy pathology reports, two indicating a higher-risk disease; the Oncotype DX score of low-intermediate risk cancer; written recommendations for surgery and brachytherapy; plus my notes from all the medical consultations.

With a good understanding of my circumstances I was able to manage and lessen the fears I had faced, specifically the outcomes that the men in the prologue experienced. What had frightened me most was an inaccurate diagnosis, to find out after treatment that I did not have cancer, as Andrew experienced. That fear was put aside. Another fear was to have begun treatment as Joe did, or to have had it completed, then to find out the cancer had metastasized, rendering the treatment unnecessary. Although that fear could not be fully resolved, I was comfortable with the prognosis that my cancer had not yet made it out onto the highway.

As for my fears of permanent, life-altering side effects, I came to view them as trade-offs. If as an outcome of warranted treatment I would have to live with one or more of them, I wanted to be absolutely certain I was choosing those over an early death. I did not want to share George's circumstances; having life-changing side effects without knowing if it were down to a choice between those or death. George is comfortable and satisfied with his decision and outcome. He wanted to rid himself of cancer and was unconcerned about the trade-offs. I respect his individual decision but do not share it.

As for my desire to find a treatment method other than surgery, as so often happens with life, we don't always get what we want. In December 2015 I selected surgery, a radical prostatectomy, the very method I'd worked so hard to avoid.

My decision was based on specific considerations. The location of my tumor at the apex and its proximity to the sphincter muscles made it difficult to achieve a clear treatment margin with external radiotherapy or HIFU, risking cancer cells being left behind. Plus, the scar tissue that would result from those methods or brachytherapy would have greatly limited the viability for surgery as a secondary treatment.

I saw two important benefits with surgery. Within weeks following the procedure I would have a very good idea of how successful it was, where with other methods it would take many long months to begin to know how successful those treatments were. Furthermore, if surgery did not remove all the cancer, I would have viable follow-up options.

The word *radical* always bothered me, so I looked it up in several sources. One usage applicable to a prostatectomy, according to *Webster*, is "designed to remove the root of a disease or all diseased and potentially diseased tissue." Although not my choice in words for this procedure, it made good sense to me. In addition to the removal of the entire prostate gland and surrounding tissues, a radical prostatectomy commonly includes the removal of seminal (semen) vesicles, sexual nerves, and some number of pelvic lymph nodes.

With the removal of the entire gland and the seminal vesicles a man will no longer be capable of sexual reproduction. With the removal of the sexual nerves the risk of erectile dysfunction is certain. The removal of many pelvic lymph nodes risks lymphedema in the legs: a condition of localized fluid retention and tissue swelling caused by a compromised lymphatic system. And there is the widely publicized side effect of incontinence to consider.

With my decision for surgery I needed a prostatectomy for sure, in that my prostate would be completely removed, but I chose a more *limited* procedure than radical meant to me. As we did not know where all the sheep were, I was not willing to extend the surgical reach deep into the lymph nodes. With the two MRIs and the three biopsy reports there was confidence that cancer had not entered my sexual nerves, so I elected a procedure that spared them. Yes, I was taking added risks, but without knowing where all the cancer was, a more limited surgery would yield a more favorable chance to protect my continence and sexual function, a quality-of-life decision.

With my treatment decision made I needed to select a surgeon. In England, doctors must make available to the public the outcomes of their procedures. There a patient can actually judge a surgeon's experience and outcomes. How empowering is that! In the United States about all we get is a postal code and the pedigrees of the fanciest medical schools and institutions known to man.

In due course I chose a surgeon close to home, Nathaniel M. Polnaszek, MD, whose staff had respectfully dubbed "Babyface." I had three consultations with him and felt he appreciated and respected my efforts and concerns. In our third consultation we discussed then agreed to remove only a few lymph nodes, to protect my sphincter muscles (to minimize the risk of incontinence), and to spare the sexual nerves entirely. I was ready to go, so we scheduled surgery for January 22, 2016.

SIX

PROSTATECTOMY AND OUTLOOK

January 2016–April 2016

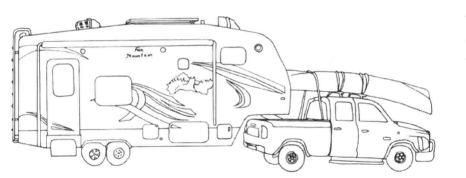

Because prostate cancer so interrupted my life and presented me with a potentially shortened lifespan, I knew I did not want to return to my business full-time. I needed a plan for post-treatment while I waited to see how successful it was.

Hiking and sailing are favorite activities of mine and I yearned for more of both. I gave much thought to sailing to exotic destinations but realized it might not be wise to be great distances from familiar medical care. So I focused on a camping trip through the Rocky Mountains, from New Mexico to Canada. Uncharacteristically for me and to my surprise—or perhaps after a change of mind—I began planning an RV road trip. The change is that in my years of tent camping I'd always scoffed at the folks in their cozy RVs. My choice was a pickup truck and fifth-wheel trailer configuration and with unexpected ease I found and purchased a used truck in excellent condition, fully configured for towing. But before selecting a trailer I had more tire kicking to do.

Surgery

Although my son Matthew is a night owl he happily drove me to the hospital before sunrise and stayed until I awoke post-surgery. When they met, Dr. Polnaszek did not hesitate to shake Matthew's deformed fingers. That was a comforting and reassuring insight to Dr. Polnaszek's character, as many people find it difficult to move past Matthew's profound disabilities.

Matthew commented that he was perfect for the robotic proce-dure, saying, *"Dad, he grew up on video games, he will do great."* What a great laugh that gave me as I was wheeled off to surgery. I was quickly prepped and positioned on the surgical table with the anesthesiologist and her assistant at my side, awaiting Dr. Polnaszek. He explained the delay—he was studying my MRIs. Feeling confident, I acknowledged that I was ready for surgical sleep.

When I woke in post-surgery recovery Matthew was there, patiently waiting. We talked for a bit and then he headed home, exhausted. I rested well. My longtime friend Dave came to visit that evening and we walked for several lengthy loops around the hospital unit. After a good night's rest I was discharged the following afternoon and Matthew drove me home. Given my condition it was a trying drive because the various drugs caused me to be very nervous and on edge. Matthew seemed to under-stand and accepted my passenger-seat-driving commentaries, which included yelling at drivers I felt were too close to our car.

Recovery

The first days home alone were very restless without the reassur-ance of the nurses that attended to me in the hospital, especially when I mistakenly thought I had broken the connector between the catheter drain tube and the urine collection bag. I made a late-night call to the duty nurse at the hospital and carefully followed his instructions to reconnect the tube. Should I ever have need for another catheter at home I will be sure to get an extra collection bag.

When the time came for the catheter's removal I was very apprehensive but that feeling was unwarranted, as it was quick and painless. Surprisingly, I immediately realized a wonderful benefit from the prostatectomy—I pee like a teenager! What I hadn't learned about was that the removal of my prostate (the enlarged dam that interfered with urination) would clear the way for unobstructed urine flow.

With recovery well under way I awaited the post-surgery biopsy report and shifted my attentions to the RV road trip. Still needing a trailer but with my physical activities I returned to online searching.

Waiting for the report was easier and less stressful than the previous times. Perhaps that was because I had a much better understanding of my circumstances and knew the report would provide a final analysis of what I had come to believe was a sheep cancer. When the extensive and detailed report was posted to my online personal patient account I focused on three details: the final Gleason score, the health of the lymph nodes, and the surgical margin.

Looking through the pages my eyes were drawn to *"Gleason Pattern and Score: 7 (4 + 3)."* That finding affirmed the concerns of the doctors in London for a more serious cancer than indicated by the first investigative core biopsy score of 3 + 3. It worried me that it was an upgrade from the second and third opinions' 3 + 4 scores.

Next, I looked for the diagnosis of the pathways for the sheep to get out onto the highway. The few lymph nodes that were removed were negative for tumor, no cancer detected but the surgical margin was *"involved by invasive cancer, focally at left apex."*

That finding of involved margin, the additional surrounding tissues that were removed with the prostate gland, was not a surprise. Going into surgery we knew the tumor location posed another pathway for spread. Recall that the MRIs indicated that the tumor was adjacent to the apex and that location was of concern to Drs. van As and Emberton with regard to their nonsurgical treatment methods for achieving clear, cancer-free margins.

During a phone conversation, Dr. Polnaszek guided me through the technical details and reassured me that the raised Gleason score was not totally unexpected. The post-surgery biopsy reflected a complete analysis of the gland, whereas the pre-surgery core biopsy was a limited view that could result in an under or overestimate of the cancer grading.

We discussed the favorable news that the final biopsy report aligned with the genomic test result and MRI reports of intermediate-risk cancer. I was finally confident my cancer was not a wolf. And with the removal of the "tumor burden," the total mass of primary tumor tissue, I had very good reason to believe my possible death from prostate cancer was pushed years out. Phew!!

But did the surgery get all the cancer? Dr. Polnaszek was concerned for the involved margin and the potential for residual cancer. He felt that even if there was residual cancer, we had good reason to believe the sheep had not gotten out onto the highway. Another phew!!

Even with the involved margin, I felt that the biopsy report validated my decisions to limit the number of lymph nodes that were surgically removed and to leave my sexual nerves intact. Without knowing where all the cancer was, I'd made a quality-of-life decision to limit the surgical reach, despite the potential risks for some residual cancer.

Testing for Remaining Cancer

Without question a prostatectomy is a major event, but it is not the final step. In actuality it is a new beginning that brings its own complications and differing medical opinions. For example, men face the reality of at least one well-published estimate—cancer remains for approximately 30 percent of men who attempt curative treatment.[18]

As with screening, following treatment, doctors and patients rely on PSA monitoring to test for the presence of any remaining cancer. Logically, with the complete removal of the prostate gland and all the cancer cells, there would be no remaining prostate antigen to measure, so the ultrasensitive PSA test is used. It measures to levels below 0.01 ng/mL. However, because a result of absolute zero is not obtainable, the term *undetectable* is used.

But what value above zero determines undetectable? This is unclear as some sources cite less than 0.2 ng/mL,[19] while others cite less than 0.1. My laboratory reports state even lower numbers: 1) *"After radical prostatectomy, the reference interval is less than 0.05 ng/mL if there is no residual disease."* 2) *"The lower limit of detection is 0.01 ng/mL."* An abstract on the National Center for Biotechnology Information website states that *"Men who achieve a nadir* (the lowest point) *of less than 0.01 ng/mL have a low likelihood of early relapse."*[20]

The definition of *undetectable* I settled on was less than 0.01 ng/mL. My first post-surgery PSA monitoring was four weeks after the procedure, which was sufficient time for all the prostate antigen to be gone by natural processes. As I had with screening, I found myself focusing on that singular result and what it meant. My test result number was 0.05 ng/mL, by some definitions a very good outcome, but I did not see it that way.

It certainly reflected the removal of the prostate gland and the tumor burden. But why was it not lower?

Although it is very unlikely, it is possible that in some surgeries a small number of healthy prostate cells could be unintentionally left behind. Those cells would continue to produce antigen—one explanation for a small amount of measurable PSA that should not increase over time. In the unwanted outcome that cancer remained, antigen would be produced by those cells. As those cells grow and spread, the PSA number will rise. More than ever I needed to manage PSA anxiety.

With my post-surgery recovery progressing I had the confidence to continue planning my upcoming RV road trip. I was excited as I looked forward to hiking, cycling, fishing, kayaking, and even backpacking. I could not think of a better way to maximize every moment, including taking a soulful look at the life in front of me and what to do if the surgery had not removed all the cancer.

Still looking for a trailer, in March 2016 I made a trip to Tucson, Arizona; its low-humidity and dry climate an oasis for quality used RVs. My brother, Brent, and his wife live there, and it was wonderful to see them. We were not close, but life can surprise us, and his interest as an uncle and his concerns for my health were bringing us together.

I made the trip to Tucson with my friend John, relying on his extensive RV experience. We visited a number of sales lots in Tucson and Phoenix before I made my purchase. For a shakedown we camped the first night near Saguaro National Park, west of Tucson. After a successful night with all systems working, we headed north into the Arizona White Mountains and then on to Zion National Park in southern Utah. With an established confidence in the rig and my new abilities with it, John

and I headed home to Austin. With just over a month to prepare the truck and trailer for my May departure back west, I had
a long list of to-dos that kept me from thinking about cancer.

SEVEN

MIRA VISTA

May-November 2016

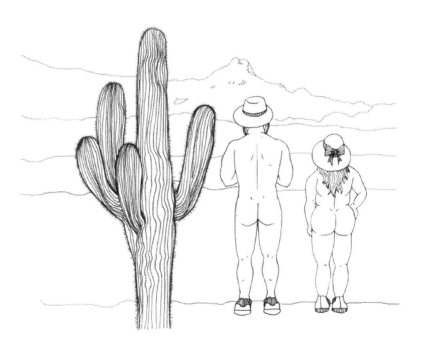

Mira Vista Resort is located on a beautiful section of land in the sun-drenched desert outside Tucson, Arizona, in the eastern shadows of Sombrero Peak. The resort's name seems to have several translations, but the one I embrace is "to see the view."

RV Camping - Season One

The start of a seven-month and nearly seven thousand-mile RV adventure is when I began writing the manuscript that evolved into this book. Throughout that trip my views and perspectives regarding cancer, treatment, and life in front of me evolved.

John, his wife Pattie, and I departed on schedule in early May 2016. They led the way in their motorhome, embarking on their eleventh anniversary of RVing. I very well remember feeling confident and grateful for my health, proud as I sat tall in my Dodge Ram 2500 3/4-ton diesel pickup truck. That hunk of powerful metal was towing my Fox Mountain twenty-eight-foot-long fifth-wheel trailer merrily along.

We had a solid travel plan for the journey, camping through the Rocky Mountains from New Mexico to Glacier National Park on the Canadian border in Montana. Our first camp was two weeks in northern New Mexico where we acclimated to mountain altitudes with hiking and cycling, then traveled into higher Colorado for June and July. We moved from campsite to campsite, exploring the mountains as the snow melted off the trails.

In early July I made a quick planned trip back to Houston to greet my new grandson, Pierce Alexander. For a week I had been on standby, waiting for the call that Shannon had delivered. The call came on the Fourth of July so the next morning I took the trailer to a nearby storage site in central Colorado, then made the long two-day drive to Houston. I can't describe how excited I was to see Shannon as a mom and to experience the joy of a newborn grandson. I spent a week supporting the family, including taking my turns at getting up at night to feed Pierce and change his diapers.

Testing for Remaining Cancer

That family-centric quick trip to Houston in July included a stop at the medical lab in Austin for my second post-surgery blood test. It was not a total shock that my PSA had increased to 0.08 ng/mL. At that moment I could have fallen into a state of depression, gloom, doom but instead with the wonderful family visit, the arrival of my grandson and a continuing road adventure in front of me, I refused to have a negative outlook.

Although a single increase did not meet insurance protocols for radiotherapy, I did ponder RT. But as I understood at that time, MRIs sensitive enough to identify the location(s) of any remaining cancer at my low PSA levels were not available, so I was not yet willing to take on the treatment. In a follow-up discussion with Dr. Polnaszek he suggested that I consult with a radiation oncologist if the third result, to be taken in November, reflected another increase.

Back to Camping

To help make the drive back to Colorado easier, my friend Dave joined me. We retrieved the trailer from the storage facility in

Buena Vista and headed to a nearby remote campsite for a few days. We then drove north to Breckenridge and met up with John and Pattie. Dave stayed a full week, then flew back to Austin from Denver. His company was appreciated, especially because I knew that cancer remained.

In August, John, Pattie and I traveled into Idaho then spent September in Glacier National Park, Montana, a favorite destination since my late teens for its spectacular beauty, abundant wildlife, and remoteness. Unfortunately, visitation is now much higher than in those days. I hope Glacier is not heading to the crowd levels I've witnessed at other national parks. Further to this concern, I am deeply saddened by the exploitation of wildlife for tourism, particularly of the grizzly bear.

We began our extended stay in Glacier on the west side of the park and moved to the east side after Labor Day. The timing of our arrival had been very carefully planned and executed. I was excited that my British friend Carole would soon arrive at the East Glacier Park Village train station. She had planned her trip from London around a brief stay in Chicago and an overnight train to northern Montana.

In early October we moved to a campsite on the western bank of the Yellowstone River, across from Yellowstone National Park. One snowy afternoon we headed into the park while most folks were leaving. Amazingly, we parked in the first public parking space at Old Faithful and had the setting nearly all to ourselves. Next we went to Grand Teton National Park but cut that visit short because of very cold wet weather and traveled south to warmer and drier Capitol Reef National Park in Utah. After two great weeks we parted paths with John and Pattie as they headed eastward, beginning their return home. Carole and I were not returning to Austin until Thanksgiving so we moved back up into the mountains in Fishlake National Forest. I had come to know the area as a teenager from Southern California and had the privilege of working there two summers for the US Department of Interior Youth Conservation Corps. What a wonderful experience that was, and fond memories brought me back.

The campground at Fish Lake was almost empty, as the late October temperatures dropped below freezing. Our closest neighbor Paul was there from Southern California for the elk hunt. We were there to cycle, hike, and fish. We found easy conversation, both being SoCal born and raised. Paul remained a Californian while I had moved to Texas when I was thirty. One evening our conversation turned to health and fitness. His father died from prostate cancer and the questions he asked were repeated by men I met throughout the trip. The lack of prostate health awareness I found during those conversations and the positive responses to my experiences further encouraged me to pursue this book.

Our next campsite was at much lower altitude with warm desert sunshine overlooking Lone Rock, Lake Powell, Utah. One morning while sitting outside the trailer enjoying a dramatic sunrise over the calm lake waters, a sudden drizzle interrupted my manuscript writing so I scrambled for cover. Reflecting on how important good health, good fitness, family, and happiness were to me I felt I had developed a sensible view of my disease. I did wonder though, without all those positive activities and connections in my life, might I have succumbed to depression, or worse, given up hope.

Leaving the warmth of Lake Powell we moved from the desert to higher elevations of the North Rim of Grand Canyon National Park, enjoying a near-empty campground and the tranquility of the mighty vistas. Each day as I hiked, biked, or exercised in another way, I knew I was maximizing my life's opportunities. We stayed for four nights, until it closed to camping on October 31, Halloween.

Months earlier I had made a reservation for the first week of November at Mira Vista resort in Tucson, which my brother manages. Although it was a two-day drive south from the North Rim, it was somewhat on the way to Austin. Our week "camping" at Mira Vista Resort presented a welcomed lens of simplicity through which to see life. The resort is clothing-optional, and while there I viewed life without the material trappings that can consume us, and without the prejudices and points of views that can cloud our thinking. Carole and I enjoyed thoughtful discussions about our countries' medical systems, based on her long successful career as an MD in England, and mine as a cancer patient. In an unexpected way that experience offered me clarity on our health care system and my responsibilities as a patient within it. In my view, the American medical industry's marketing of cancer as a "fight" or "war" is incongruent with patient-centric health care and each patient's harsh realities with this disease.

85

The highlight of the visit with my brother and his wife was a simple celebration of his birthday, since we must have been in our teens when we last celebrated a birthday together. Leaving Mira Vista, Carole and I drove southeast to Big Bend National Park in southwestern Texas, along the border with Mexico. Arriving at the park entrance we reflected that Carole had joined me in Glacier National Park at the Canadian border, some two thousand miles north of where we now were.

To celebrate the end of the RV journey, Matthew, Shannon, Kyle, and my grandson, Pierce Alexander, made the long drive from Houston to join us for a short stay in Big Bend. We had a wonderful visit in the vastness and isolation of Big Bend. One morning Kyle and I took the Boquillas ferry, a very brief row-boat ride, from the official US Port of Entry within the park to the Mexican town of Boquillas del Carmen on the other side of the Rio Grande. There we met Señor Chalo Díaz who offered his services as a personal guide. Appreciating that he likely made a good part of his earnings this way, we welcomed his company. We had fun discussions over lunch including the election of Donald Trump. Chalo shared that Mexican friends of his living in the States had voted for Trump—and that Trump's victory was welcomed by the locals. One desire they had was that the "wall" would stem the flow of illegal drugs into the United States, and thereby diminish the reign of terror caused by the cartels in Mexico. Learning of their reality has left a lasting impression on me.

Because Carole was interested in seeing Boquillas, she and I took the ferry over for lunch and to shop for a miniature copper wire tree that Matthew had seen for sale along a hiking trail. The residents of Boquillas sell their crafts at honesty-box displays along hiking trails in the park to raise monies for their family and the community. Chalo was on the bank and eagerly joined us for lunch then helped us look for a miniature, but none were to be found—so he offered to make one. We agreed on a price, shook hands, and made arrangements to meet the following day.

That next morning I rose for a pre-sunrise walk heading for the bank crossing on the Rio Grande to meet Chalo. The November 14, 2016, supermoon was setting in the west behind the Chisos Mountains and there was a slight chill in the air. It seemed as if the birds were singing, saluting the rising sun as I heard Chalo singing right along with them. As he walked out of the lush tall grasses that lined the river's edge we saluted each other and then forded the knee-deep waters, meeting in the center of the river. The tree he made matched my description well; Matthew would be pleased.

Our stay at Big Bend ended the day campsite reservations began, the official start of the winter camping season. To break up the long hard haul to Austin we enjoyed a brief layover on Lake Amistad, about the halfway point.

Back home my first order of business was a visit to the GP's office for my third post-surgery PSA test. In anticipation of the outcome and with Carole's assistance I researched post-surgery radiotherapy.

Some Reflection

I remain amazed at the sheer variety and volume of opinions and options that are available to prostate cancer patients, but I think there might be even more regarding RVs. I stepped inside well over fifty carefully selected trailers before making a purchase. Then prior to departure I shopped extensively for add-on features including a solar power system, a battery inverter, and a stand-alone portable heating unit. My experience with health care research also paid off in my quest for an excellent RV.

For example, the treeless campsite on the shore of Blue Mesa Reservoir, west of Gunnison, Colorado, provided abundant sunlight for the solar panel to charge and maintain the rig's batteries, a frugal alternative to the gas-powered generator. Each morning I did strengthening exercises and yoga, guided by workout videos I brought along. Several evenings I watched favorite movies and indulged in long, hot showers. Not once did I have to start that noisy generator. Things changed though when I moved to the forested mountains surrounding Twin Lakes, on State 82, between Leadville and Aspen.

The campsite is a popular base camp location for Mount Elbert, the highest peak in Colorado at 14,440 feet above sea level. On the first morning there, my well-insulated Fox Mountain fifth-wheel kept me warmer than the tent campers around me, but temperatures inside still dropped to the upper fifties. Before working on the manuscript, I turned on my portable propane heater. That awesome little *Mr. Heater* was a great alternative to the rig's furnace, which runs a power-hungry fan, and it was essential at a location like Twin Lakes where the solar panel was shaded by pine and aspen trees, and where cloudy skies were common. In those situations, solar generation is very limited and battery power must be conserved. Using the propane heater not only conserved battery power, but also precluded the need to heat the rig with the gas generator.

As with many things, I like to have different approaches and options to choose from. Rather than accept the standard RV offerings, I researched adaptations and made additions to suit my requirements. That is how I approached and continue to approach my prostate cancer.

EIGHT

RADIOTHERAPY AND OUTLOOK

December 2016-October 2017

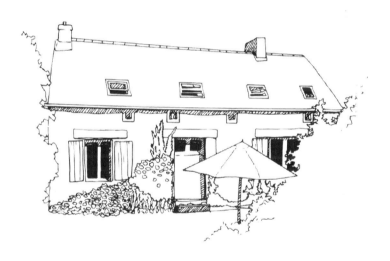

As a patient I found the consideration of post-surgery radiotherapy a gray area of uncertainty. For circumstances such as mine, when only a small amount of cancer remains, it did not seem possible for current science to identify precisely how much there was or where it all might be. That led to the question—could RT get it all?

Treatment right after surgery is commonly called *adjuvant (auxiliary) radiotherapy* and is done in attempt to kill suspected or known cancer that surgery could not reach and remove. Treatment following a post-surgery PSA rise, indicating cancer remains, is commonly referred to as *salvage radiotherapy*. Neither term worked for me, as they felt at best, misleading. From my perspective, I was considering life-extending radiotherapy treatment.

Recall that my first post-surgery PSA monitory test was higher than we wanted, indicating that cancer possibly remained. Then the second test, during my quick trip to meet my grandson, reflected a slight increase. The third, taken the week of Thanksgiving 2016, was another unwelcomed increase.

Carole and I had a comfortable, open discussion with Dr. Polnaszek, who suggested I meet with a radiation oncologist. He recommended Douglas J. Rivera, MD, for radiotherapy treatment. An appointment with Dr. Rivera was readily available, and fortunately, Carole was able to join me before she returned to England.

I knew what I was looking for in a doctor, and Dr. Rivera was spot-on. We began a useful and trustful conversation straightaway about the reliability and meaning of my rising PSA. His feeling was that cancer had spread into the barnyard, before the prostatectomy. I asked if my body's immune system could naturally eliminate the remaining cancer cells. He said it was possible, but that it was also possible for the remaining cells to become wolves. I asked what he thought the progression would be; he felt that my PSA would continue to rise as the cancer spread. At the end of the consultation a blood sample was drawn; it showed another upward tick. Graph 3 reflects that rising trend.

Graph 3: Rising PSA Following Surgery

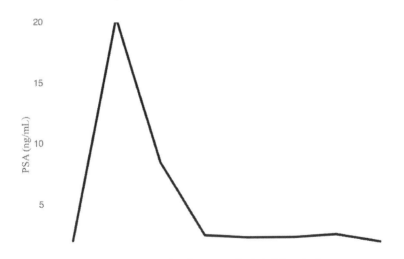

Note: My nadir (lowest point) 0.05 ng/mL

The big question was how far the small amount of remaining cancer had spread. In other words, where were all the remaining sheep? If RT hit all the cancer cells, there was every reason to believe they would be killed: a curative outcome. However, if cancer cells had spread beyond the reach of RT, they would not be killed: a noncurative outcome.

The best investigative tool available to detect where all the cancer is is imaging. Dr. Rivera had experience with a newer imaging method, the fluciclovine PET CT, but he did not feel even it was sensitive enough to detect my small amount of remaining cancer. Although it was not covered by insurance, I did consider self-paying for the scan. But given that it was unlikely to identify any suspicious sites, I did not have it done because I did not want to waste time and money on unreliable hope.

Even though my PSA was low and it was unlikely that imaging could identify any of the remaining tumor(s), I decided to go forward with localized radiation treatment to the prostate bed. Although there was rationale for treatment to a larger area of the pelvic region, I was not willing to risk tissue and organ damage without knowing for sure that I was choosing between those trade-offs and an early death. I felt the same way when I decided to limit the surgical reach of the prostatectomy, and I remain comfortable with both decisions.

Treatment Regimen

My schedule of thirty-nine RT sessions started before the New Year 2017 rang in. As the treatment process would take nearly eight weeks to complete, I felt I needed another project, a diversion, something to put positive energy into. One of my hobbies is refurbishing boats; it brings real pleasure and a sense of accomplishment to take a boat that is not suitable for use and return it to a useful purpose. Taking on such a project when I was "fighting" for my own longevity seemed like a great idea, so

I did a quick search and found a project: a 1970 Mako 17 fishing boat. I had always been a fan of older Mako center-console fishing boats, and now I had my own to work on. Other than needing fresh paint and bit of electrical work, the boat was in good shape. It was a perfect find, and I set the goal of finishing the work before my radiation treatments were completed. My thinking was to work on the boat after my morning radiation sessions. What a beneficial project that was! In my experience, no matter how positively one approaches adjuvant/salvage radiotherapy, it is damn difficult to get through the months of treatment.

In preparation for RT, I had an MRI of the prostate bed and a CT scan of the pelvic area. Additionally, a leg mold was made and pencil-tip-sized tattoos were applied to the target area to aid precise body positioning on the radiation machine table. I never wanted a tattoo, but under the circumstances, I made an exception. A medical team then reviewed the pertinent records along with the new scans to determine optimal beam placement for radiation and dosages. During the sessions, I got a glimpse of that amazing science. Software process sequences were displayed on the monitor above the radiation table as the computer guided the machine through its steps, including automatically adjusting radiation targeting and dosages.

Each of the thirty-nine days of radiation followed the same routine. While driving to the facility each day, I drank twelve ounces of water to ensure that my bladder was full. Never having to wait long after my arrival, I was warmly greeted and walked through secure doors to the radiation chamber. I would dress down in the changing area and then the team of technicians positioned me on the radiation table. They would maneuver me back and forth a bit by pulling on the sheet

94

beneath me, aligning my pelvic tattoos with the lights on the radiation machine. When things were all set, they cheerfully left the room, shutting the radiation-shielded door behind them. Next was a quick scan to make sure my bladder was adequately full. As the noisy radiation process began, the machine made multiple 360-degree passes around me. The treatment sequence took only a few minutes to complete.

Overall, my experience was routine and without drama or difficulty. Late in the second week, I faced several days of serious exhaustion and a bout with nausea, but that was all I endured. To this day I think of the patients I saw during RT who did not fare as well as I did. It was difficult to know what to say, how to feel.

Because the RT treatment process went so well, I had a surgical hernia repair straightaway. The hernia occurred near my navel, a primary entry point for the robotic method used for the prostatectomy. The hernia was not caused by the surgery, but rather was a result of the condition known as diastasis recti. *Diastasis* means "separation," and *recti* refers to the abdominal muscles called the rectus abdominis. When the left and right abdominal muscles separate, a thin band of connective tissue remains. That is where the hernia pushed through, at the surgical entry point.

Apparently, the condition is not uncommon for women after pregnancy, and men also get this type of hernia, possibly from doing sit-ups or weightlifting improperly or yo-yo dieting. I've never yo-yo dieted, but whatever the cause of my hernia, I was happy to have it repaired. My thinking was to use the coming months for dual recovery from hernia surgery and radiotherapy.

After radiotherapy I was back to the question of whether treatment had gotten all the cancer. PSA testing would provide the answer. The general recommendation is to wait a good number of months before testing to allow sufficient time for prostate cancer cells to die from the exposure to radiation. We decided to wait four months.

Les Marchais

Instead of anxiously waiting at home for the months to pass, I planned a fun-packed trip back to Europe. Besides, I was nearly sixty, so celebration was in order. In mid-March, three weeks after the completion of RT and the hernia repair, I packed my bags and was off for a three-month adventure with friends to see and places to go.

My first stop was Dorking, where I stayed at the Waltons. As that trip was put together on short notice, I was quite lucky to be able to see friends. A highlight of the visit was that I helped Maggie and Richard slow-cook a brisket on their brand-new American-made Big Green Egg, a ceramic kamado-style charcoal grill. I must say that brisket was as good as any I have ever had in Texas.

With a beer in hand and a plate full of charcoal-cooked brisket, I was asked about my dietary choices, especially given my cancer. What a challenging and personal subject. With so many books and opinions, where does one start? My simple answer was that throughout my adult life I have always eaten what I believed was a healthy diet, including limited amounts of meat. Even though I was facing cancer, I was not ready to radically change my eating habits. I did not see a change in diet as a means to a cure.

My next adventure was March skiing with Carole in Zermatt, Switzerland, a bucket list item. Ever since I saw a movie about it in high school, I have wanted to climb the Matterhorn. As it was the winter season, I had to settle for gazing upon the iconic mountain. With the best of good fortune, we arrived at the tail end of a significant snowfall and the beginning of a full week of excellent weather. After a wonderful week of skiing, we took a restful train ride through the Alps to visit with my friends Peter and Delores from Dorking at their home in Chamonix, France. Peter and Delores were wonderful hosts and we so enjoyed our brief stay with them.

We departed Chamonix by train for Carole's new home, a two-hundredish-year-old stone farmhouse within the Parc Naturel Regional in Normandie-Maine in western France. Carole's ambitious plan was to open a bed-and-breakfast before the summer holiday season. Many French country homes are named and the historical name of Carole's is Les Marchais. One translation is "the walk", perhaps because the property abuts long established pilgrimage routes. (The illustration preceding this chapter is of Les Marchais.)

Prior to welcoming guests, we had a lot of work to do. We started ripping out parts of every room, including all the doors and frames. We took down and replaced several insulating walls that had been laid over the original stone. Digging into the stone and clay walls that were made by bare hands one rock at a time provided a look into how people built their homes hundreds of years ago. We took a chance and sandblasted paint off the large granite fireplace that once served as the original cooking center, revealing beautiful stone. With careful planning we installed a modern kitchen.

Fortunately, we had the fine assistance of a skilled builder, and occasionally other skilled workers as well. The beautiful walled garden required a massive effort to reclaim it from unchecked vegetative growth. The large multiroom barn needed a major clean-out as well. In addition to hard work, my principal skill was wall painting, or *decorating*, as the Brits call it. I acquired that skill through a teenage job and continue to enjoy it.

Those months of physical work were a wonderful way to continue my physical and psychological recovery from RT and the hernia repair. Putting new life into a declining structure was more than a metaphor; it was what I was trying to do for myself. I got physically stronger each day, and my spirits were elevated by our daily progress with the renovations. We wrapped up the work on the house in early June. Carole was ready for her first guests, and I returned to Austin.

98

Testing for Remaining Cancer

It had been four months since the completion of the radiotherapy, so I went straight to the doctor's office for the first blood test upon my return to Austin. Despite how great I felt, my anxiety over the success of the radiation treatments had mounted. That anxiety was warranted; the reduction in PSA was much lower than expected. We had the same question as when my first post-prostatectomy test was not as low as expected. Despite an attempt at curative treatment, the result indicated that cancer remained. The next test would provide further information, but that would not be for another six months.

RV Camping - Season Two

In addition to getting the RV ready for the upcoming summer and fall road trip, I made several visits to Houston to see my daughter, her husband, and my grandson. And with beautiful June weather, I enjoyed sailing *On Edge* and fishing on the boat I had refurbished during the RT treatments.

I joined up with John and Pattie, who I traveled with the previous year, in late June. After several weeks in Colorado we went north to Grand Teton National Park because we'd had to cut short our visit there the year before due to inclement weather. We then moved into Idaho to find a relatively quiet campsite for the upcoming August 2017 "Great American Eclipse." Wow, that experience certainly exceeded expectations, and we enjoyed watching the entire event from our campsite. After an extended stay in Idaho, we headed south to Great Basin National Park in Nevada, then east into Utah, and returned to Capitol Reef National Park.

In mid-September John and Pattie moved eastward while I remained in southern Utah for several weeks concentrating on fishing then headed southwest toward Las Vegas. Carole joined me there from France for the remainder of my 2017 RV adventure. After a brief stay in Nevada's Valley of Fire State Park, we went to Death Valley National Park; an amazing first experience for both of us.

Leaving Death Valley, we headed southwest into the Mojave Desert south of Mount Whitney. My longtime friends Steve and Holly lived on a nice piece of land there with unobstructed views of the mountains. It was an easy park of the trailer, and we enjoyed a week-long visit with them. We had experienced amazing changes in landscape, from the lowest point in Death Valley to Mount Whitney in the High Sierra. Carole walked among Joshua trees and giant redwoods, both must-sees of hers. At the end of our wonderful visit with Steve and Holly we headed west to the Pacific Coast, another first-time experience for Carole.

NINE

BETWEEN A ROCK AND A HARD PLACE

November 2017-March 2018

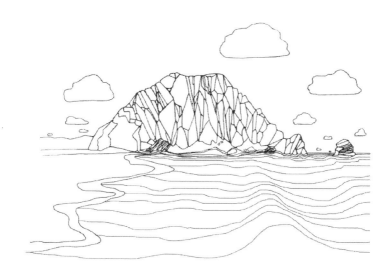

opened the second chapter with an illustration of my sailboat *On Edge* and wrote about feeling that way during my years with screening. I continue to feel that way with PSA monitoring for remaining cancer post-treatment. In November of 2018, nearly two years after the prostatectomy and ten months after the RT, many factors brought on a new feeling: that of finding myself between a rock and a hard place.

Carole and I were RV camping along the beach in Morro Bay, California, where from our campsite we enjoyed a good view of Morro Rock, a volcanic mound in the bay. I was in continued good health and fit from another summer of wonderful hiking, trail running, and cycling. It was unplanned on my part, but we happened to be camping within a short walk of the athlete transition area for the upcoming Morro Bay Triathlon, which had open registration. What a fun way to continue to bring in my sixtieth year. I felt the urge to sign up, but the lingering effects of a mountain bike crash months earlier back in Idaho forced me to pass on the opportunity.

I settled for quiet walks and jogs along the surf, kayaking in the bay, and an occasional bike ride. By happenchance we were the fifth and sixth persons to sign up for whale watching, meeting the minimum passenger requirement for a three-hour excursion. With six guests and the captain onboard and no other boats in sight, we had an exceptional experience watching gray whales up close. We also enjoyed the bayside fishing village for fresh seafood delights, regional craft brews, and tunes by local musicians.

Camping at Morro Bay provided another opportunity for both reflection and looking forward. It had been three years since DRE screening identified the lesion on my prostate gland. Since then, my skills as a patient detective, patient scientist, and self-advocate had become well developed. But I began to question whether my efforts had served me well. My early screening proved to have been the correct thing to do, but we missed the warning signs. Despite all the hope, the prostatectomy did not remove all the cancer, so I tried RT. But the first post-radiotherapy test raised doubt. One morning while jogging toward Morro Rock, it hit me. I was between a rock and a hard place. If the upcoming PSA blood test result was not down but up, indicating that cancer remained and was growing, what was I going to do?

Although I wanted to stay longer, we left before the triathlon to begin the drive back to Austin. To make the long-haul easier, we stopped in Tucson to visit with my brother and his wife. As we had the previous year, we camped in luxury at Mira Vista Resort.

The morning after our arrival at Mira Vista I made a visit to a local medical clinic in Tucson and the next day I had my answer. My PSA had not gone down; it was up. I was grateful to Carole for being there and we had several extensive discussions on the issue. Was the small rise simply a variance in laboratories—and not an indicator that cancer remained? Was it an error? Or was it a sure sign that cancer remained? We attempted to chill out in the warm fall sunshine for a few more days then began the long drive to Austin for Thanksgiving with my family, plus a scheduled consultation with my radiation oncologist.

Oh Bollocks, Again!

Dr. Rivera was open and honest as we discussed the obvious: my cancer had spread beyond the reach of the radiotherapy before the treatment and it was growing. In my words, the sheep had gotten out of the barnyard. Despite the conclusion that I faced microscopic cancer in the pelvic region, there was good to be cherished. My health and fitness remained great, so we had worthy cause to continue believing that my cancer was not a wolf and that the onset of symptoms from distant organ metastasis was a long time off.

Recall that before RT we'd considered the fluciclovine PET CT imaging technique but decided against it because Dr. Rivera did not think it was sensitive enough for my low PSA level and my health insurance did not cover it. With a rising PSA post RT, we looked into whether coverage had become available, and for another data point to submit to the insurance company, we did a third blood test; as shown in graph 4, another uptick.

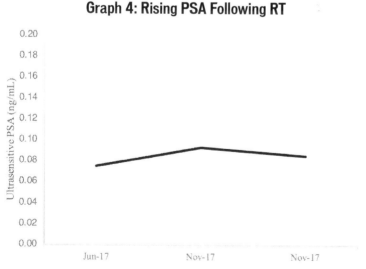

Graph 4: Rising PSA Following RT

Note: My nadir (lowest point) 0.075 ng/mL

Starting from the first post-RT blood test result of 0.075 in June 2017, the November numbers, 0.091 and 0.083 respectively, indicated a subtle rising trend. The first and third tests were analyzed by the same laboratory in Austin. The second was from the Tucson clinic, taken just weeks earlier while visiting with my brother and his wife. A plausible explanation for the second value being slightly higher than the third is that the Tucson clinic used a different laboratory.

Although my insurance company declined to cover the fluciclovine PET CT, they offered the less sensitive choline PET CT—but I would have had to travel to Arizona or Minnesota. I found myself in another hard-place moment. Either travel considerable distance at my expense for the "less sensitive" choline PET CT my insurance covered, or self-pay for the "more sensitive" fluciclovine PET CT that most likely would still not be sensitive enough for my circumstances. In subsequent email communications with Drs. Rivera and Polnaszek, Dr. Polnaszek advised of an even newer technique, the PSMA PET CT. Unfortunately, it was not available in the US outside research settings, and health insurance wasn't covering it in late 2017. With strong evidence that my cancer remained, and with no assured means to find it, I was discouraged.

A side note: in the same week that my insurance provider declined coverage for the more sensitive imaging technique Dr. Rivera suggested, they approved full coverage for my sixtieth-year colonoscopy, including the preparation kit. This is evidence of the disconnect between the lack of standardized screening for prostate cancer, which kills more men than colon cancer, and insurance companies' readiness to fully cover colon cancer screening.

That Patient Detective, Patient Scientist, Self-Advocate Thing

When I crashed the opening reception party at the September 2016 World Molecular Imaging Society's conference in the Grand Tetons, I could not have imagined that just over a year later I would be seeking the most advanced imaging technique available for my critical need. Through additional research I came to fully appreciate that the forward-looking and progressive Europeans were leading the way with imaging. Turns out the PSMA PET CT was standard practice in Europe. The fluciclovine PET CT, which my insurance company had declined to cover, and the choline PET CT, which my insurance approved, were already considered older technologies there.

Carole's contacts in England proved invaluable. Networking led me to Professor Anwar R Padhani, an internationally recognized oncological MRI radiologist in London. He thought my PSA indicated remaining cancer. Although he offered a PSMA PET CT or a PET MRI (*"maybe slightly better"*) at the London Clinic, he recommended a PSMA PET CT combined with nanoparticle MRI.

After reading about that mouthful of imaging technology, I asked Professor Padhani for the referral. Turns out, the nanoparticle MRI was only available from Radboud University Nijmegen Medical Centre—in the Netherlands. With an upcoming winter trip to England and France, going there was feasible and reasonable.

Nanoparticle MRI in the Netherlands

Opening an email dialogue with Jelle Barentsz, professor of radiology and chairman of the Radboud University Nijmegen Prostate MR Center of Excellence, was easy. After reviewing all the information, I grasped how involved the procedures would be; they would require two days to complete. In an email exchange, I asked what the outcome would be if the procedure did not identify any sites suspicious for cancer. His answer was that at a minimum I would have an excellent baseline for future reference. My thinking was that, just as with a negative biopsy, not finding cancer with the most advanced imaging available did not render the procedure unnecessary. From my perspective, no suspicious findings would strongly indicate that very few and very small sheep remained.

Even though it would be an expensive self-funded investigation, I knew I wanted to give it a try. Before selecting my next treatment method it was imperative for me to know the location of my remaining tumor(s). With the formal acceptance of my submittals, the procedures were scheduled with Professor Barentsz at Radboud University for early January 2018. Even though Nijmegen was an eight-hour drive from Carole's home, driving proved easier than taking the train or flying.

The university hospital was less than three miles from our hotel, so Carole and I decided to walk. Northern Europe is very cold and dark at 0800 in January, so we bundled up. With flashlights in hand we hopped over patches of ice along the paths in the woods while the locals peddled by on their bikes, undaunted by the cold and dark.

Soon after our arrival at the hospital I was given an IV infusion of nanoparticle contrast medium; fine bits of iron that were referred to as "the black stuff." This was done first because the black stuff needed to circulate for twenty-four hours before the procedure. The IV drip was administered with the personal care of Professor Barentsz and took over an hour to complete, providing an opportunity for very interesting discussions.

For the upcoming PSMA PET CT, a radioactive saline solution was machine-infused into my other arm while I sat alone in a special shielded room. I was instructed to stay a safe distance from children and pregnant women for the next twenty-four hours; I was not quite sure what to think of that.

After the infusion I was escorted to the imaging center for the PSMA PET CT. The procedure confined me to the tunnel scanner for about an hour. Afterwards, Carole and I walked several miles in good late-afternoon weather from the university campus to the center of Nijmegen, Holland's oldest city. We found our way to the medieval Grote Markt square and dined in a pub located within a Renaissance building that had survived the bombings of WWII. That was a fun way to end an otherwise long and taxing day. After our return to the hotel, I quickly went to sleep, looking forward to the next day's big event: the nanoparticle MRI.

The procedure was scheduled for the afternoon, and we considered a morning drive to a nearby war museum, but ultimately decided not to risk being late for the procedure. I instead enjoyed a leisurely swim and sauna before our midday walk back to the hospital. After check-in we went straight to the imaging center. To my surprise, I was a bit of a celebrity with the medical staff, being from Texas and all. Plus, our walks from the hotel were not their idea of typical American behavior; we are known from TV and movies as drivers of big cars, not walkers. The technicians asked about the *Wild West* and wondered if I rode horses, so we shared some good laughs. As it had the day before, the procedure confined me in the tunnel scanner for an hour. Halfway through, shots were administered into each leg, but rather than stress I simply made jokes with the technicians.

After the procedure Carole and I went back to Grote Markt square. Rather than walk we opted for the bus. At the start of dinner, I began to feel quite ill. It seemed my blood pressure crashed—perhaps in part because I drank a beer on an empty stomach. I was about to get sick, so the pub staff happily packed our meals to go and put us in a taxi back to the hotel. I slept through the night, awakening some fourteen hours later. Well rested, Carole and I made the long drive back to her home.

Sheep at the Checkpoints

January is very cold in northwest France, and there was nothing heartwarming about the nanoparticle MRI having identified five lymph nodes suspicious for cancer.

> *Level of Suspicion (LOS): 1=benign; 2=probably benign; 3=equivocal; 4=uncertain malignant; 5=malignant*

> *There are three suspicious nodes (LOS 4), right pelvic (obturator fossa and presacral). There are two equivocal nodes (LOS 3). There are no signs for bone marrow metastases.*

> *Radiologic Impression: 5 potential positive nodes, not positive on the PSMA-scan due to the small size.*

The finding of no signs of bone marrow metastases was a major relief; it supported the hope that my cancer remained localized to the pelvic region, in lymph node checkpoints but not out on the blood vessel highway.

The fact that the potentially positive nodes were not identified on the PSMA PET CT scan validated my expenditures for the nanoparticle MRI, for it is critical to appreciate the ramifications regarding the sensitivity of the various imaging techniques. The PSMA PET CT scan, despite being standard in Europe, was just becoming available in the USA in 2018. How grateful I am that through networking I found my way to Professor Barentsz. And how I worry for the men that do not have access to such investigative technology.

Treatment Consultations

The most difficult and frustrating period for me as a patient self-advocate was when I had the nanoparticle MRI results in hand. I knew full well that few doctors had experience with this investigative tool and I had no expectations that my insurance company would approve treatment based on the unfamiliar MRI.

Back at Carole's home in France, I continued researching treatment options. Extensive reading and multiple consultations presented radiotherapy, hormone therapy, and chemotherapy as the principal methods for salvage lymph node treatment. Surgery, it seemed, was not a common option.

Radiotherapy to the larger pelvic region risks permanent bowel issues due to tissue scarring, as well as lymphedema resulting from damage to the pelvic lymph nodes. Hormone therapy has its own basket of trade-offs. Although I understood that chemotherapy does not have permanent trade-offs, it would be a tough six months of treatment. Further adding to my reluctance was my understanding that these methods were generally for latter-stage cancers, and not deemed curable treatments. Once again, I weighed quality-of-life risks against morbidity.

Continued research on the web opened up the possibility for surgery. Specifically, it was this statement in a medical publication from the European Association of Urology titled *Salvage Lymph Node Dissection in Recurrent Prostate Cancer Patients.*[21]

> *Surgically removing pelvic and/or retroperitoneal lymph nodes that were visible in one or two locations on [11C] choline PET/CT [4] introduces a new concept of salvage lymphadenectomy* (the surgical removal of lymph nodes) *in patients with low biochemical PSA recurrence.*

What boosted my confidence was that the nanoparticle MRI was a far more sensitive technology than the choline PET/CT cited in that paper, which was published back in 2011. What troubled me was that the choline PET/CT was the very method my insurance company approved in late 2017. That raised the question: Just how far behind is American prostate cancer health care?

I reached out by email to my surgeon and oncologist in Austin, plus several other American doctors I was referred to. No one suggested the nanoparticle MRI findings should be discounted or ignored, but I received no immediate clear answers. After a bit of frustration, I realized that I might have to travel back home to meet with the doctors in their respective offices; I was uncertain as to what I might learn.

While I was focused on medical research, Carole had been looking at ski reports, as the January 2018 snowfall was exceptional. She found several bargain ski-in/ski-out accommodations. Without hesitation we booked a week in Flaine, France, packed our ski gear, and jumped in the car.

In additional to having great ski days and wonderful evenings, we both continued our research. One evening while browsing technical papers online, Carole came across Professor Dr. Alexandre Mottrie, head of the urology department at OLV Ziekenhuis Hospital in Aalst, Belgium.

I remain amazed at how easily one can access doctors in Europe, and how much information about their careers is publicly available. After extensive reading by both of us, I sent Professor Mottrie an email with my nanoparticle MRI findings. Here is his prompt reply: *"Dear sir, I am actually in the Alps as well. I propose salvage lymphadenectomy robotically. We can call on Tuesday if you want. Sincerely, Prof dr Mottrie."*

As offered, I called Professor Mottrie while taking a break from skiing. Unfortunately, he was not available as a surgery had come up so the call was rescheduled. To my pleasant surprise I received his return call the next evening. That conversation began a flow of communications and Professor Mottrie offered to conduct a full review of my nanoparticle imaging.

After Flaine we made the short drive to Chamonix to visit and ski with my friends Peter and Dolores, as we had the year before. We then made the long drive back to Carole's house, using that time to go over our notes and discuss treatment options, giving serious consideration to surgery with Professor Mottrie.

For one additional datum I went to Carole's GP for a PSA test, which revealed another upward tick. With four measurements I had no doubt my PSA was rising. During a phone consultation with one American doctor he suggested I have a third test back at the Austin facility to avoid variations in laboratory testing. I gave that some thought, but concluded the additional assurance was unnecessary.

Yes, I had results from three different laboratories: ones in Austin, Tucson, and France. And maybe, with testing at these

113

extremely low levels, one billionth of a gram, slight variations between laboratories is possible. But does it matter? Whichever combination of my results is graphed, even with such close values, it indicates an upward trend from the first test.

More definitive than a rising PSA level were the nanoparticle MRI results. For me, those findings trumped all concerns regarding measurements from different laboratories. I was convinced additional treatment was warranted, and soon. But which treatment method?

Despite what seemed like a lack of support for extended lymph node dissection, to my thinking surgery still offered the benefits I'd appreciated when I selected the prostatectomy. If surgery successfully removed all (or nearly all) the cancer, within a few weeks my PSA would be undetectable: the ultimate objective. If that did not occur, at the least I would have the pathology report, providing more definitive conclusions on the MRI findings and my remaining cancer.

With those perspectives and knowing that Professor Mottrie is a world-class leader in this surgical technique, I accepted his confident recommendation and scheduled surgery for early March, 2018. Twenty-six months had passed since my prostatectomy. I wondered if, when, and how my treatment journey with prostate cancer might end.

Salvage Lymphadenectomy in Belgium

As Carole and I made the long drive to Aalst, I was comfortable and relaxed. I had no concerns about being away from home and American doctors. I knew surgery was the best treatment decision for me, and that I was going to perhaps the best surgeon in the world for my specific procedure. However, that reality seemed quite surreal, for I had strived to ignore all the messaging and marketing about finding the best doctors and treatment centers. I wish to note I never saw one medical services billboard in Europe.

The medical facilities I experienced in Europe operate much like ones in America, or perhaps vice versa. Although English was adequately spoken at the hospital, I did appreciate that their principal language was Dutch, and that I was having surgery in a foreign country. So, to make things easier I hired a medical service agency. They provided translations when needed and guided our movements through pre-admissions procedures and pre-surgery testing. Additionally, they arranged for an extended hotel stay for my initial recovery period and transportation to and from the hospital. That service by Betamedics Premium Medical Agency proved more helpful and valuable than I had anticipated. I was glad I spent the additional monies.

As I went into the afternoon surgery, I had a good understanding of the procedure strategy, which I will attempt to share in patient speak. Professor Mottrie would remove the common left and right iliac lymph nodes, which are grouped along the common iliac artery, a major checkpoint. They would be immediately biopsied and diagnosed by the frozen section procedure, taking only minutes. If cancer was identified in those lymph nodes, Professor Mottrie would then extend the surgical reach to find and remove as many pelvic lymph nodes as possible, in an attempt to remove all the cancer in the pelvic region. If cancer was not found in the common iliacs, the surgery reach would not be extended to further pelvic lymph nodes; rather it would focus on the nodes going back to the prostate bed.

It was late evening when I awoke from what I later learned was a long procedure. I recall being very groggy and confused.

The nursing staff was excellent, and with their help I had a comfortable night's rest.

Professor Mottrie came to see me early the next morning. He explained that the lymph node dissection procedure was extensive. Cancer was found in the common iliacs. I was immeasurably grateful for Professor Mottrie's skills and his surgical strategy. Remaining significant tumor burden was removed, and perhaps all the cancer. Later that morning Carole came to visit. She brought me treats and stayed for the afternoon. We concentrated on positives including the exciting news that Shannon had given birth to my second grandchild while I was in surgery. I rested very well that night knowing I was in good health and would be back in Texas soon seeing my family, and my granddaughter, Alanna Jade, for the first time.

Feeling very good on the second morning following surgery, I was discharged from the hospital on the condition that I would stay at a hotel in nearby Ghent for a week. While I was recovering at the hotel, each day Carole and I did short walks around the historic city center, enjoying the medieval architecture, the twelfth-century Gravensteen Castle, and a few Belgium beers. What a wonderful way to recover.

Biopsy Report

After a week of good recovery, we returned to the hospital for a post-surgery examination and to meet with Professor Mottrie. He had just received the report and took us through it. A total of thirty-one lymph nodes were removed. Six were found to be metastatic. Some might say six is a lot. I maintain the view that twenty-five were free of cancer.

Following a very favorable post-surgery examination I was fully discharged. Feeling strong, confident, and optimistic, I flew home to Austin the next day. The only sad part was saying goodbye to Carole.

Testing for Remaining Cancer

The morning after my arrival home I went to my GP to have blood drawn. Although ten days post-surgery is insufficient time for all of the antigen to be removed from my body, I needed an indication as soon as possible. Recall that my first PSAs after the prostatectomy and subsequent RT had not gone down as much as we had hoped. Testing at ten days would provide a good projection of the treatment outcome.

I was alone, in my home office, when the report arrived by email. The same desk my daughter sat at when she received her acceptance email from Johns Hopkins University. When Shannon opened her email, she sang out with enthusiasm. When I opened the report online I stared and stared. Then I read out loud: "0.03 ng/mL" I could not have been more excited. I could not have been more relieved. By many medical accounts that's undetectable. Some would say cancer-free!!

I planned to have the next (second) blood test on the twenty-fourth day after surgery. Despite my excitement and a countdown calendar on my refrigerator, I was casual about going to the GP's office, and arrived too late in the afternoon for blood testing. As it was a Friday, I had to wait until Monday for the blood draw and several more days for the result. A self-inflicted delay.

Oh my, was the wait worth it! The result: less than 0.01 **ng**/mL. By all medical accounts, that's undetectable for prostate cancer. Immediately I called Carole. When she answered, I shouted with great emotion, "Less than 0.01, less than 0.01, less than 0.01!" Happiness abounded, as there could be no better outcome.

The findings of Professor Barentsz's nanoparticle MRI and the outcome of Professor Mottrie's subsequent surgery resulted in my prostate cancer being undetectable. Although I knew better than to think I was cured, I was and remain very jubilant and optimistic.

Hormone Drug Therapy

Since cancer is a lifelong journey, this amazing success represented yet another beginning and another hard place. Did this third treatment get all the cancer? PSA was undetectable in my blood, but we have no absolute assurance that all the cancer is gone. If I still have cancer, there is no means of determining where all those sheep are hiding. It will take many years of testing to know for sure, so is wait and see all I can do?

There is developing scientific reason to believe that if cancer remains, it is probably still in the pelvic region, and the optimal time to treat it, attack it, is when it is undetectable. So again I found myself considering radiotherapy to the pelvic region, hormone therapy, and chemotherapy. And as before, I weighed quality-of-life risks against morbidity. With considerable thought and anguish I decided against the radiotherapy and chemotherapy, not yet willing to take on the trade-offs without absolute certainty that cancer remained.

Not wanting to simply wait and see, I found a reasonable compromise—daily hormone drug therapy. Although it may not be necessary, if it is, the goal is to delay or even stop any remaining cancer cells from dividing. I realize that if I still have cancer I should not depend on hormone therapy as a curative treatment. However, if undetectable cancer remains, and this therapy buys me more years, then I may well die of something else even though prostate cancer lies in wait. That is an outcome and a statistic I can live with.

Despite the trade-offs being extensive, intimidating, and even frightening, they should ease once treatment ends. And because I can choose to stop treatment at any time I have daily control. The list includes: allergic reactions, high blood sugar, high blood pressure, various infection-like symptoms, shortness of breath, significant weight gain, swelling in arms or legs, enlarged breasts, breast pain, change in urination, chest pain, muscle weakness, severe tiredness and weakness, deadly liver or lung problems. The list goes on to include hot flashes, unwanted hair growth, nausea, diarrhea or constipation, ED, dizziness, sleepiness, excessive sweating, back/pelvis/stomach pain, headaches, anxiety. Hoping to offset possible breast pain and enlargement, I had a session of radiotherapy to my breasts.

From the long list of possible scary side effects I experience only a few. These are shortness of breath, breast pain, uncharacteristic tiredness, hot flashes, and nausea. Additionally, my libido has taken a full hit. I am also dealing with weight gain, although I must admit it's partly because my activity levels are down but my caloric intake is not. Although partially bald, I am growing new and longer hairs elsewhere but dealing with this trade-off by enhancing my skills with scissors and a body hair trimmer. Perhaps worst of all is the gynaecomastia—better known as the onset of man boobs. As a direct result of the testosterone-blocking drug, a hormone imbalance has my ratio of estrogen to testosterone leaning to the female side.

RV Camping - Season Three

Consistent with my plans the previous two years, I was back in my RV for the 2018 camping season. I wanted an easier pace this time, though, as I had concerns for my risks of lymphedema from the lymphadenectomy, and I was apprehensive about the side effects of the hormone therapy.

So I decided to spend most of the season camping in one place, at an easier pace. With this in mind I took the responsibility of camp host at the semiprimitive Pettit Lake Campground in the Sawtooth Mountains of Idaho. I had visited the area in my two previous RV journeys and wanted to explore the mountains more extensively. As the campground has only twelve sites, I felt the hosting responsibilities would be a fair trade-off for the privilege of camping in such a beautiful place for the camp host season, running from May to mid-September 2018. My hope was to fully regain my strength and fitness while enjoying the lake, forests, and mountains. With a bit of luck I would be fit enough for a triathlon; perhaps the Morro Bay California triathlon that I passed on last year.

In June, with my PSA anxiety well under control, I drove twenty miles from my campsite to the Salmon River Clinic in the remote mountain town of Stanley for my next test. My greatest hope was realized: another sub 0.01 ng/mL reading, still undetectable for cancer. Then, just before my duties ended in September I went to the clinic for my six-month test. With great relief and satisfaction, the result was again undetectable for cancer. Whether the undetectable status is a sole result of the lymph node removal surgery or of the added hormone therapy doesn't matter to me. I am just grateful for the outcome and for what is surely a long delay in my possible death from prostate cancer. And, just maybe, I am cured of prostate cancer.

After my campground hosting duties were over I joined up with my friends John and Pattie and spent a few weeks more in Idaho, then moved on to Utah for an extended stay. With early snows and cold temperatures looming we headed farther south into New Mexico. After a week's stay in the warmer desert climate, John and Pattie began their trek home to Austin while I made a swing westward to Mira Vista Resort in Arizona to visit my brother and his wife. We capped our visit with a hike up Sombrero Peak (the illustration for Chapter 7, Mira Vista).

As for my hope for a triathlon, I passed on last year's because of a bike crash but this year I was just not fit enough. Needing an excuse, I blamed the hormone drug therapy. It was a fair trade-off for enhanced chances of being cancer free.

At the end of my 2018 RV season I returned to Austin for a complete physical with my GP, including the nine-month post-lymphadenectomy blood test. My PSA continued to be undetectable for cancer and since all other aspects of the physical examination were within normal, healthy parameters and guidelines, I received a clean bill of health. With such good news I gave thought to stopping the daily hormone therapy but decided to continue on with it, perhaps for up to two years total if my PSA remains undetectable. That time frame is based on evidence that if a man's PSA remains undetectable for cancer after two years, his continued outlook for being prostate cancer free is very good.

Thanksgiving 2018

Even more wonderful than the good health news was Thanksgiving with Matthew, Shannon, Kyle and my grandchildren, Pierce and Alanna. In addition to wonderful family visits, I enjoyed a bit of sailing aboard *On Edge* and some fishing on the Mako power boat I refurbished during my RT sessions. Soon thereafter I headed back to Dorking, England to stay with Richard and Maggie of the Waltons, and to visit with friends.

Then off to Les Marchais, Carole's home in France, for the 2019 ski season. And of course, the next rounds of ultrasensitive PSA blood tests with her GP.

THE BRIDGE

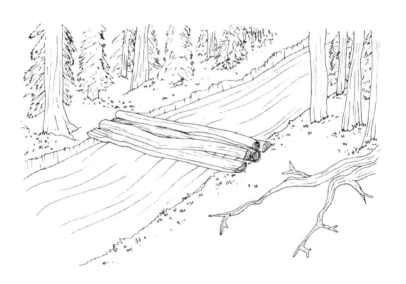

H uman health and bridges can be fickle. When I was diagnosed with prostate cancer and realized my self-directed screening had failed me, it felt as if the rug had been pulled out from under me.

I experienced that feeling early into the 2016 RV trip on a hike with my friend and RV'ing buddy John.

We began our hike at the 9,000-foot trailhead register on the upper West Fork of the Conejos River, which flows from the San Juan Wilderness in southern Colorado to the Rio Grande River southwest of Alamosa. It was amazing to be in such a beautiful place experiencing such good health so soon after cancer surgery.

Two backpackers had signed the register a few days earlier and identified themselves with the only other car in the parking area. A few miles in we entered the San Juan Wilderness and came upon the fork in the trail we were looking for. The right fork headed up Roaring Gulch to Bear, Twin, Timber, and then Glacier Lakes, but we opted for the left fork which appeared to have less snow and continued along the stream which was about twelve feet wide and looked to be up to waist deep. The fast-moving water was rough and boiling due to large rocks and tree debris so if one fell or got a leg stuck while trying to cross, the situation could get deadly serious.

Soon we crossed paths with the two backpackers and their dogs hiking out. They shared trail information and the location of a log bridge they had hastily constructed farther upstream.

Thanking them, we continued onward and found the bridge they spoke of, five felled trees cleared of branches spanning the bank. The logs were loosely bundled and not tied together or even anchored at the ends.

Without fear or hesitation John quickly crossed the bridge and reached the other side. I was hesitant and pondered the primitive structure but had to admit that John and the two heavily laden backpackers had already tested it.

With John on the other bank I ventured onto the bridge, right foot, left foot, right foot, left foot, right foot, CRACK! CRACK!! Splash, splash, splash!!! Suddenly another *oh bollocks!* in my life—the logs under my right foot snapped like toothpicks and fell into the waters below. I instinctively dropped the hiking pole in my right hand since continuing to lean on it would have taken me into the frigid waters. Still standing I was balanced only on my left foot firmly planted on one of the remaining three logs while my right foot dangled above the waters below. Calm, collected, and in control I slowly crept backward to the safety of the bank.

John came back across the broken bridge and we looked in vain for the hiking pole but we never discussed my close escape. One moment the bridge to the other bank of the stream looked safe. It had supported the three others but as I walked across logs broke unexpectedly beneath my feet. I did wonder, had I come close to being another man with prostate cancer that died from another cause?

During my years of prostate cancer screening I was healthy and active, feeling safe with the widely published statistic that three out of four men with an elevated PSA do not have prostate cancer.[22] Then unexpectedly I was the one out of four men

126

whose elevated PSA was because of cancer. My bridge had broken.

John and I sat down to a brief lunch. Afterward he crossed the bridge again to explore the other side. I decided to explore the side I was on. I walked in the forest giving thought to where I was— emotionally in the wilderness of prostate cancer. I was grateful that the surgery and recovery had gone so well, that I was fit and able to take long strenuous hikes at high altitudes. And I was grateful I survived the bridge.

Life was good and I was maximizing every moment. What is important for me and my continued health is to maintain that attitude in my lifelong journey with cancer.

.

ACKNOWLEDGMENTS

I would like to express my thanks to my editor, Stacey Donovan, whose wisdom and experience helped turn this raw and sometimes inconsistent story into a cohesive narrative. Also, much appreciation to my review team. Anna Wyatt is an aspiring editor/publisher who helped me in the beginning. Stacy Formby and her husband, Steve, provided great insights prior to editing. And my friend Al Schwerman offered brilliant final reviews and suggestions.

A multidisciplinary medical approach is not standard practice in the United States so I sought medical professionals I was comfortable with. My confidence in my therapeutic pathway would have been impossible without the informal medical team I was able to assemble. I am deeply grateful for my practitioners (listed alphabetically): Dr. Nicholas van As, The Royal Marsden, London, England; Professor Jelle Barentsz, Radboud University, Nijmegen, the Netherlands; Professor Mark Emberton, University College Hospital, London, England; Michael J. Hilts, MD, Scott & White Healthcare, Georgetown, Texas, USA; Professor Dr. Alexandre Mottrie, OLV Hospital, Aalst, Belgium; Mehul K Patel, MD, Baylor Scott & White Clinic, Round Rock, Texas, and Assistant Professor, Texas A&M College of Medicine, Bryan, Texas, USA; Nathaniel M. Polnaszek, MD, Assistant Professor of Surgery, Baylor Scott & White Healthcare,

Round Rock, Texas, USA; Douglas J. Rivera, MD, Austin Cancer Centers, Austin, Texas, USA; and last but not least, Mr. Sarb Sandhu, consultant urological surgeon, New Victoria Hospital, London, England.

APPENDIX A

WHAT I WOULD TELL MY BROTHER

D ispel the misinformation that prostate cancer is an old man's disease; that screening has unmanageable risks; and that men should fear overtreatment and unwarranted side effects.

Appreciate that more men would die from this disease if they did not die from something else, sooner (a dunk in a freezing mountain stream comes to mind).

Take responsibility for the decisions, actions, and inactions regarding your prostate health. Follow through with regular screenings and be mindful that even with normal PSAs and DREs, cancer may be present. Consider graphing your PSA results and be attentive to even the slightest upward trend.

Imaging (currently MRI or ultrasound) should be performed if any concern is identified. Give careful thought to the degree of sensitivity you want to rely upon—for imaging techniques are not created equally.

If a biopsy is recommended, quell all fears and appreciate that they are a walk in the park compared to childbirth (or so they say). Request imaging to target the biopsy needle to the more concerning areas of the tumor to obtain a better analysis of the cancer threat. Consider a second reading of the biopsy pathology, because critical decisions are based on the grading.

If cancer is diagnosed, obtain a genomic assay (or something similar) to help determine the risk of the tumor.

Consult with an independent oncologist to determine whether the cancer is a sheep or a wolf, and when possible determine if it is localized to the barn, the barnyard, or out on the highway.

Seek as many opinions as required to determine the best treatment plan, including consultations with professionals who will not be performing your treatment.

Medical research papers, although technically daunting do provide clarity and consensus on the newest developments in screenings, investigative methods, and treatments. Well-conducted studies reflect independent thinking free of marketing influences.

Always be chasing! Whether I was seeking information, appointments, medical records, biopsy slides, or a reply, I found it necessary to chase after them all. If not, valuable time is lost while you wait unnecessarily, adding to the anxieties one already faces.

Maintain detailed notes of your various body and health functions. Once you begin treatments, it is difficult to recall exact details about your life functions such as sleep, energy, urination, and bowel movements. Don't worry about your body temp or your blood pressure since nurses will record these ad nauseum.

With the current turmoil in our health care system a solid medical savings plan is essential, adding to it whenever possible.

Recognize that cancer is a lifelong journey, and that there is no assurance of early detection or a sure cure.

Have a good sense of your lifestyle values and maintain physical and mental fitness.

APPENDIX B

ABOUT CONTINENCE

U rinary incontinence and bowel function regularity are common fears of men diagnosed with prostate cancer. Fortunately, I do not have significant continence issues. In addition to my skillful surgeons I give credit to the daily Kegel exercises I did prior to and after surgery. This is not to say things are perfect. Occasionally I do dribble. There are times when I unintentionally release urine, especially when I wait too long and get up from a seated position. Doing Kegel exercises just prior to these situations seems to help, except when I have consumed alcohol.

During one of my discussions about the risks of radiation tissue damage to the bladder, the doctor referenced the line "never trust a fart" from the movie *The Bucket List*; a story about men dealing with cancer. Over time I have come to understand this sentiment. Although my bowel regularity is good I am still cautious and do wonder if I will experience a change. Even if a change occurs, it may be merely because of aging and not the treatments.

APPENDIX C

ABOUT ERECTILE DYSFUNCTION (ED)

Because I was concerned about the impact surgery would have on my sexual function, despite the risk of leaving some cancer behind I elected to have a sexual-nerve-sparing prostatectomy. For six months after the procedure I could not achieve an erection. Then I began to recover naturally, although not enough for intercourse. The pleasure of orgasms returned, but without ejaculate, because the body parts that produce that fluid were removed. I was not frustrated with the situation because it seemed a fair exchange for ridding my body of cancer and it was better than an early death. Although I did consider ED medication, I choose instead to allow more time for full, natural recovery.

Just over a year after the nerve-sparing prostatectomy, and despite RT to the prostate bed, I began experiencing natural erections firm enough for intercourse. With those successes and after additional thought, I tried ED medication. It helped occasionally, but not always. I am grateful that as I age into my sixties having had prostate surgery and RT, I am able to achieve satisfactory sexual function and orgasm naturally.

When I started the hormone drug therapy I was well informed on the many trade-offs, including ED. Although my libido has taken a full hit, I do expect this to be corrected when I stop taking the drug.

APPENDIX D

REPRESENTATION OF MALE PELVIC AREA

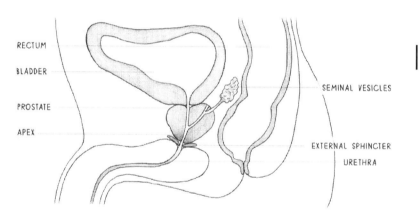

RECTUM

BLADDER

PROSTATE

APEX

SEMINAL VESICLES

EXTERNAL SPHINCTER

URETHRA

AUTHOR'S NOTES

Please note that this is not a medical book, nor should it be considered self-help. This book stories my quest as a patient to try to avoid the outcomes of the other men in the prologue.

I wrestled with the inclusion of personal experiences, not because they are a secret but because you, the reader, might not have any interest. The reality, though, is that without family, friends, and fun diversions, I might have rushed into treatment, or worse, gone into denial. So I've included what I hope you find to be helpful and inspiring personal tidbits. I also wrestled with the inclusion of the illustrations, and after much thought kept them in with the rationalization of author's prerogative. And besides, I really like them.

My Objectives with This Book

1. To debunk the landslide of misinformation concerning prostate cancer and vigorously challenge the widespread misconception that it is an old man's disease.
2. To relate the story of how I went from diligent screening at the age of forty-one to ignoring warning signs because of misinformation; and to share what can be done to avoid making the same errors.

3. To rattle the cage of those who claim that American health care is best in the world.

If I can achieve part of these objectives, my fumblings in writing this book will have been more than worthwhile.

ABOUT THE AUTHOR

Murray was a very healthy and active young man, not predisposed to prostate cancer and not in a high-risk category due to family histories, race, or old age, who came to have prostate cancer.

He is an average man's man, leaving home at eighteen and supporting himself ever since. He has a zest for life while being a humble, discreet man. Murray is a father of two and raised them on his own from elementary school onward. His daughter, Shannon, graduated from Johns Hopkins with honors in neurology, then earned her PharmD from the University of Texas. His son, Matthew, has established considerable independence despite his severe disabilities of being armless, handless, and legally deaf while living with kidney disease.

Murray has always wanted to write, but until his experience with prostate cancer he had not found the topic or the necessary passion. He was a successful small IT business owner with offices in the US and UK. He stepped away from the business at fifty-eight to pursue his health options and to maximize every minute of life, including the writing of this book.

His next book, anticipated to be published in 2020, is about the incredible struggle of living with severe disabilities in America—as experienced and as seen through the eyes of a loving, committed father.

ENDNOTES

1. Reported in Cancer Research UK (website), "Statistics by Cancer Type," (London, 2017), accessed September 2018, http://www.cancerresearchuk.org/health-professional/cancer-statistics/statistics-by-cancer-type.

2. Hashim U. Ahmed, Ahmed El-Shater Bosaily, Louise C. Brown, et al., "Diagnostic Accuracy of Multi-Parametric MRI and TRUS Biopsy in Prostate Cancer (PROMIS): A Paired Validating Confirmatory Study." *The Lancet* 389, no. 10071 (February 25, 2017): 815–822, accessed September 2018, https://www.thelancet.com/journals/lancet/article/PIIS0140-6736(16)32401-1/fulltext.

3. Quoted in James Gallagher, "Huge Leap in Prostate Cancer Testing," BBC News Online, January 20, 2017, accessed September 2018, http://www.bbc.com/news/health-38665618.

4. H. Ballentine Carter, *Prostate Disorders: Your Annual Guide to Prevention, Diagnosis, and Treatment* (Berkeley, CA: University of California School of Public Health, 2018). H. Ballentine Carter, MD, is professor of urology and oncology and the director of adult urology at the Johns Hopkins University School of Medicine. Available from: https://www.healthandwellnessalerts.berkeley.edu/white_papers/prostate_disorders_wp/UCB_WHP_C_landing.html, accessed September 2018.

5. Otis Brawley, "Epidemic of Overtreatment of Prostate Cancer Must Stop," CNN Health website, July18, 2014, accessed

September, 2018, http://www.cnn.com/2014/07/18/health/pros-tate-cancer-overtreament/index.html.

6. Reported in Centers for Disease Control & Prevention website, "United States Cancer Statistics, 2015 Top Ten Cancers", accessed September, 2018, https://gis.cdc.gov/Cancer/USCS/DataViz.html.

7. Reported in American Cancer Society website, "Key Statistics for Prostate Cancer," (Atlanta, Georgia, 2017), accessed February 2018, https://www.cancer.org/cancer/prostate-cancer/about/key-statistics.html.

8. *2017 Prostate Disorders: Your Annual Guide to Prevention, Diagnosis, and Treatment*, page 33.

9. *2017 Prostate Disorders: Your Annual Guide to Prevention, Diagnosis, and Treatment*, page 34.

10. *2017 Prostate Disorders: Your Annual Guide to Prevention, Diagnosis, and Treatment*, page 33.

11. United States Preventative Services Task Force (USPSTF), draft recommendation statement "Prostate Cancer: Screening" May 8, 2018, accessed October 2018, https://www.uspreventiveservicestaskforce.org/Announcements/News/Item/final-recommendation-statement-screening-for-prostate-cancer.

12. Canadian Task Force on Preventative Health, published guidelines on prostate cancer in Neil Bell, Sarah Connor Gorber, Amanda Shane et al., "Recommendations on Screening for Prostate Cancer with the Prostate-Specific Antigen Test." *CMAJ* 186, no. 16 (November 4, 2014): 1225–1234, accessed September 2018, https://canadiantaskforce.ca/guidelines/published-guidelines/prostate-cancer/.

13. Public Health England, "Prostate Cancer Risk Management Programme (PCRMP): Benefits and Risks of PSA Testing," (London, 2016), accessed September 2018, https://www.gov.uk/government/publications/prostate-cancer-risk-management-programme-psa-test-benefits-and-risks/prostate-cancer-risk-management-programme-pcrmp-benefits-and-risks-of-psa-testing.

14. Reported in University College London (website), "Prostate MRI Scans Increase Cancer Detection & Reduce Overdiagnosis," (London, 2018) accessed September 2018, http://www.ucl.ac.uk/news/news-articles/0318/190318_prostatebiopsy.

15. The definition of *pathology* is from the *English Oxford Living Dictionaries* online, accessed September 2018, https://en.oxforddictionaries.com/definition/pathology.

16. *2017 Prostate Disorders: Your Annual Guide to Prevention, Diagnosis, and Treatment*, page 44.

17. Genomic Health, Inc. announces "Medicare Establishes Final Local Coverage Determination (LCD) for Use of the Oncotype DX® Genomic Prostate Score™ Test in Patients with Favorable Intermediate-risk Prostate Cancer Effective October 9, 2017," accessed September, 2018, http://investor.genomichealth.com/releasedetail.cfm?releaseid=1038123.

18. *2017 Prostate Disorders: Your Annual Guide to Prevention, Diagnosis, and Treatment*, page 51.

19. *2017 Prostate Disorders: Your Annual Guide to Prevention, Diagnosis, and Treatment*, page 50.

20. National Center for Biotechnology Information, "Ultrasensitive Serum Prostate-Specific Antigen Nadir Accurately Predicts the Risk of Early Relapse after Radical Prostatectomy." *The Journal of Urology* 173, no. 3 (2005): 777-80, accessed September 2018, https://www.ncbi.nlm.nih.gov/pubmed/15711268.

21. Arnulf Stenzl, "Salvage Lymph Node Dissection in Recurrent Prostate Cancer Patients." The European Association of Urology, DOI of original article: 10.1016/j.eururo.2011.07.060, 935943, accessed September 2018, https://www.europeanurology.com/article/S0302-2838(11)00895-5/abstract.

22. The James Buchanan Brady Urological Institute, Prostate Cancer Update, Volume VI, winter 2003, accessed February 2018, http://urology.jhu.edu/newsletter/prostate_cancer64.php.

Made in the USA
Columbia, SC
03 June 2020